Dena Shenk, PhD
Lisa Groger, PhD
Editors

Aging Education in a Global Context

Aging Education in a Global Context has been co-published simultaneously as *Gerontology & Geriatrics Education,* Volume 26, Number 1 2005.

Pre-publication
REVIEWS,
COMMENTARIES,
EVALUATIONS . . .

"**O**FFERS A WEALTH OF INFORMATION, RESOURCES, AND GUIDELINES for teaching cross-cultural gerontology and for the worldwide promotion of gerontological and geriatric education. The book is filled with model course designs, class projects, pedagogical strategies, and suggestions for the enrichment of classes through the use of international film and literary works that focus on late life. The book also advances the state of gerontological education worldwide by providing models for international academic teaching and research partnerships between the United States and developing countries. It is HIGHLY RECOMMENDED AS ESSENTIAL READING FOR GERONTOLOGICAL EDUCATORS with interests in global aging."

Margaret A. Perkinson, PhD
Research Associate
Washington University in St. Louis
Editor-in-Chief
Journal of Cross-Cultural Gerontology

"**C**OMPREHENSIVE. . . . A VALUABLE RESOURCE for all who have an interest in the field of aging, cross-cultural issues, and globalization. This book offers both breadth (aging education, globalization, cross-cultural issues) and depth (course design and content development on thanatology, literary portrayals of elders, and cinematic approaches to cross-cultural teachings). Many mediums are represented–health care practice, service delivery, international partnerships, and institutional curriculum development. Each chapter contextualizes the issues associated with aging and globalization, providing a compelling foundation for integrating these topics into gerontology education. Select chapters provide strategies and/or resources to enhance cross-cultural content and teaching in aging."

Marilyn R. Gugluicci, PhD
Director
BodyWISE Center
for Health and Fitness
Assistant Professor
Department of Family Medicine
University of New England
College of Osteopathic Medicine

"**O**ffers a global perspective on aging that is ESSENTIAL TO ALL GERONTOLOGICAL EDUCATORS. Christine Fry's chapter, 'Globalization and the Experiences of Aging,' serves as a helpful primer on the effects of globalization before directly addressing its impact on older persons. Most useful in helping to explain these effects are the three anecdotal examples Fry provides from Africa, Canada, and the United States. The book also includes two unique examples of how educators might integrate cross-cultural experiences into courses on aging. It also offers rare insight into the status of gerontological education in Kenya and Japan."

Rona J. Karasik, PhD
Director, Gerontology Program
and Professor of Community Studies
St. Cloud State University, Minnesota

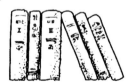

More Pre-publication
REVIEWS, COMMENTARIES, EVALUATIONS . . .

"**I** HIGHLY RECOMMEND THIS PUBLICATION FOR INSTRUCTORS AND LEARNERS who are focusing specifically on gerontology content, or for learners and instructors in disciplines such as social work, sociology, or psychology, where the content can be infused as part of a course. Readers are presented with an understanding of the core principles of cultural diversity and then are given examples of resources that can be used to infuse cultural diversity issues related to aging and intergenerational concerns throughout an existing course. These resources can also be used to develop specific courses in aging. The book also provides some insight into how gerontology educational programs here in the United States are being used as models for teaching gerontology in other countries."

Catherine J. Thompkins, PhD
BSW Program Director
Department of Social Work
George Mason University

"**G**ERONTOLOGISTS, ANTHROPOLOGISTS, SOCIOLOGISTS, HEALTH EDUCATORS, AND OTHERS WILL BENEFIT FROM THIS WORK. It will not only serve as a reference for issues in a graying world but also as a source to spur others to venture outside their discipline to explore gerontology through the eyes of others."

Kathy Segrist, PhD
Gerontology Program Director
Fisher Institute for Wellness
and Gerontology
Ball State University

"**P**ROVIDES IMPORTANT PERSPECTIVES, methodologies, and Internet resources to help us understand the future of aging education within Western and non-Western cultures."

Howard R. Gray, PhD
Professor and Coordinator
of Academic Internships
Brigham Young University

More Pre-publication
REVIEWS, COMMENTARIES, EVALUATIONS . . .

"FRESH. . . . UNIQUE. . . . AN INVALUABLE FONT OF NEW IDEAS AND STRATEGIES for successfully bringing our students into the increasingly globalized world in which they live and work. It is often difficult to create a coherent and consistently well-written volume from conference proceedings. However, the co-editors have done that and more. The scope and disciplinary reach of the authors and perspectives explored are truly impressive. Contributions draw from the fields of anthropology, sociology, literary criticism, film studies, religious studies, gerontology, and social work."

Jay Sokolovsky, PhD
Professor
Division of Arts and Sciences
University of South Florida

The Haworth Press, Inc.

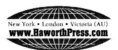

New York • London • Victoria (AU)
www.HaworthPress.com

Aging Education in a Global Context

Aging Education in a Global Context has been co-published simultaneously as *Gerontology & Geriatrics Education*, Volume 26, Number 1 2005.

Aging Education in a Global Context, edited by Dena Shenk, PhD, and Lisa Groger, PhD (Vol. 26, No. 1, 2005). *"Provides important perspectives, methodologies, and Internet resources to help us understand the future of aging education within Western and non-Western cultures." (Howard R. Gray, PhD, Professor and Coordinator of Academic Internships, Brigham Young University)*

Cultural Diversity and Geriatric Care: Challenges to the Health Professions, edited by Darryl Wieland, PhD, MPH, Donna Benton, PhD, B. Josea Kramer, PhD, and Grace D. Dawson, PhD (Vol. 15, No. 1, 1995). *"Provides a wide variety of perspectives on caring for a growing diverse elderly population. The content is broad and applicable to many cultures because the authors manage to keep clear of stereotypical classifications and offer theoretical frameworks and some practical strategies that may apply in numerous situations." (Social Work in Health Care)*

Geragogics: European Research in Gerontological Education and Educational Gerontology, edited by Celia M. Berdes, MSPH, Adam A. Zych, PhD, and Grace D. Dawson, PhD (Vol. 13, No. 1/2, 1993). *"Reviews the previous and current research in the two overlaps between gerontology and education, with much emphasis on the methodologies of the emerging discipline." (Reference & Research Book News)*

Death Education and Research: Critical Perspectives, by W. G. Warren, MA (Vol. 9, No. 1/2, 1989). *"A very thought-provoking and thorough overview of the theoretical background of the many complexities concerning death education and research." (Oncology Nursing Forum)*

Aging Education in a Global Context

Dena Shenk, PhD
Lisa Groger, PhD
Editors

Aging Education in a Global Context has been co-published simultaneously as *Gerontology & Geriatrics Education*, Volume 26, Number 1 2005.

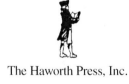

The Haworth Press, Inc.

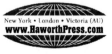

New York • London • Victoria (AU)
www.HaworthPress.com

Aging Education in a Global Context has been co-published simultaneously as *Gerontology & Geriatrics Education*™, Volume 26, Number 1 2005.

Cover design by Kelly E. Fye

Library of Congress Cataloging-in-Publication Data

Aging education in a global context/Dena Shenk, Lisa Groger, guest editors.
    p. cm.
    "Co-published simultaneously as Gerontology & geriatrics education, Volume 26, Number 1 2005.
    Includes bibliographical references and index.
    ISBN-13: 978-0-7890-3080-1 (hard cover: alk. paper)
    ISBN-10: 0-7890-3080-2 (hard cover: alk. paper)
    ISBN-13: 978-0-7890-3081-8 (soft cover: alk. paper)
    ISBN-10: 0-7890-3081-0 (soft cover: alk. paper)
    1. Gerontology. 2. Aging–Study and teaching. 3. Geriatrics–Study and teaching. 4. Aging–cross-cultural studies. I. Shenk, Dena. II. Groger, Lisa. III. Gerontology & geriatrics education.
HQ1061.A42485 2005
305.26'071–dc22   2005203771

Indexing, Abstracting & Website/Internet Coverage

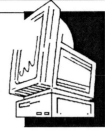

This section provides you with a list of major indexing & abstracting services and other tools for bibliographic access. That is to say, each service began covering this periodical during the year noted in the right column. Most Websites which are listed below have indicated that they will either post, disseminate, compile, archive, cite or alert their own Website users with research-based content from this work. (This list is as current as the copyright date of this publication.)

(continued)

(continued)

Special Bibliographic Notes related to special journal issues (separates) and indexing/abstracting:

- indexing/abstracting services in this list will also cover material in any "separate" that is co-published simultaneously with Haworth's special thematic journal issue or DocuSerial. Indexing/abstracting usually covers material at the article/chapter level.
- monographic co-editions are intended for either non-subscribers or libraries which intend to purchase a second copy for their circulating collections.
- monographic co-editions are reported to all jobbers/wholesalers/approval plans. The source journal is listed as the "series" to assist the prevention of duplicate purchasing in the same manner utilized for books-in-series.
- to facilitate user/access services all indexing/abstracting services are encouraged to utilize the co-indexing entry note indicated at the bottom of the first page of each article/chapter/contribution.
- this is intended to assist a library user of any reference tool (whether print, electronic, online, or CD-ROM) to locate the monographic version if the library has purchased this version but not a subscription to the source journal.
- individual articles/chapters in any Haworth publication are also available through the Haworth Document Delivery Service (HDDS).

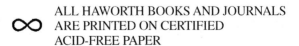

Aging Education in a Global Context

CONTENTS

ABOUT THE EDITORS

Dena Shenk, PhD, is Director of the Gerontology Program and Coordinator of the Graduate Program at the University of North Carolina at Charlotte, where she is Professor of Anthropology. Her primary research interests are diversity within the older population based on gender, culture, and environment with an emphasis on individual expectations and experiences of aging. Her recent publications include *Someone to Lend a Helping Hand: Women Growing Older in Rural Minnesota, Teaching About Aging: Interdisciplinary and Cross-Cultural Perspectives*, and articles in the *Journal of Cross-Cultural Gerontology, Aging and Identity*, the *Journal of Women & Aging, Ageing and Society*, the *Journal of Aging Studies*, and *Educational Gerontology*. Dr. Shenk was the elected Chair of the Commission on Age and Aging of the International Union of Anthropological and Ethnological Sciences (ICAES) from 1998 to 2003, is a Fellow of the Gerontological Society of America, and a charter Fellow of the Association for Gerontology in Higher Education (AGHE) and the UNC Institute on Aging.

Lisa Groger, PhD, is Professor of Gerontology and Director of Graduate Studies in Gerontology at Miami University in Oxford, Ohio. Her research has focused on African Americans' informal support networks and care-giving issues. Her work has appeared in the *Journal of Cross-Cultural Gerontology, Journal of Aging Studies, International Journal of Aging and Human Development, Journal of Aging and Ethnicity, Journal of Applied Gerontology, Human Ecology, Research on Aging*, and *Qualitative Health Research*. She has contributed to a number of edited volumes, including a chapter, with Jane Straker, on combining qualitative and quantitative methods in gerontology for the Second Edition of *Qualitative Gerontology*. Dr. Groger serves on the editorial board of the *Journal of Aging Studies* and has previously served as Treasurer for the Association for Anthropology and Gerontology (AAGE).

Introduction:
Aging Education in a Global Context

Dena Shenk, PhD
Lisa Groger, PhD

SUMMARY. Introduction to a collection of articles on aging education in a global context based on the proceedings of the annual conference of the Association for Gerontology in Higher Education (AGHE). The volume includes a dual focus on (1) issues related to gerontology and geriatric education around the world, and (2) issues related to teaching about global and cross-cultural aging. Several of the chapters provide useful information and resources for educators seeking ways to incorporate cross-cultural aging into their courses. The remaining three chapters deal with issues related to aging education in Kenya, Japan and China. *[Article copies available for a fee from The Haworth Document Delivery Service: 1-800-HAWORTH. E-mail address: <docdelivery@haworthpress.com> Website: <http://www.HaworthPress. com> © 2005 by The Haworth Press, Inc. All rights reserved.]*

KEYWORDS. Global aging education, cross-cultural aging, aging education, Kenya, Japan, China

---

Dena Shenk is Director, Gerontology Program and Professor of Anthropology, Department of Sociology and Anthropology, University of North Carolina at Charlotte, 9201 University City Boulevard, Charlotte, NC 28223-0001 USA (E-mail: dshenk@email.uncc.edu).

Lisa Groger is Professor, Department of Sociology and Gerontology, Miami University, Oxford, OH.

[Haworth co-indexing entry note]: "Introduction: Aging Education in a Global Context." Shenk, Dena, and Lisa Groger. Co-published simultaneously in *Gerontology & Geriatrics Education* (The Haworth Press, Inc.) Vol. 26, No. 1, 2005, pp. 1-7; and: *Aging Education in a Global Context* (ed: Dena Shenk, and Lisa Groger) The Haworth Press, Inc., 2005, pp. 1-7. Single or multiple copies of this article are available for a fee from The Haworth Document Delivery Service [1-800-HAWORTH, 9:00 a.m. - 5:00 p.m. (EST). E-mail address: docdelivery@haworthpress.com].

Available online at http://www.haworthpress.com/web/GGE
doi:10.1300/J021v26n01_01

As anthropologists who study aging, we are both committed to incorporating a comparative approach to aging into our teaching. We were pleased to have this opportunity to develop a volume encompassing some of the work being done in global aging education. Interest in global aging has increased dramatically out of necessity, as several of the contributors to this volume note in their chapters. Three of these developments were outlined in the introduction to the third edition of *Teaching About Aging: Interdisciplinary and Cross-Cultural Perspectives* (Shenk and Sokolovsky, 1999). These include first, the enormous burst of research and publications on aging in non-Western cultures as well as ethnic groups in North American and European contexts. A second change has been the growth of a qualitative and cross-cultural approach to aging beyond the disciplinary bounds of anthropology that has been referred to as "qualitative gerontology." A third very dramatic change is the availability of educational resources through the internet. These changes have continued during the intervening years since that volume was published.

This volume is being published by Haworth Press in a special arrangement with the Association for Gerontology in Higher Education (AGHE) as the partial proceedings of the 2004 AGHE annual conference. The book is being published simultaneously as a special issue of the journal of *Gerontology & Geriatrics Education.* Haworth Press invited us to co-edit a special publication of the journal from the Proceedings of the annual conference because of its focus on global aging; thus most of the papers were first presented at that meeting held in Richmond, Virginia, February 26-29, 2004. The theme was "Globalizing Gerontology and Geriatrics Education" and the charge was to think about how we can make a positive difference on a global scale. Every nation is confronting the ethical, economic, social, and political dilemmas that aging populations present. Neither American gerontologists nor those in other countries can afford to remain unmindful of the aging of people around the globe, for we have much to learn from each other about how aging is changing every nation and how those changes will transform the world we inhabit.

The volume includes a dual focus on (1) issues related to gerontology and geriatric education around the world, and (2) issues related to teaching about global and cross-cultural aging. Several of the chapters provide useful information and resources for educators seeking ways to incorporate cross-cultural aging into their courses. These include the chapters by Fry, Elliott, Nandan, Yahnke and Waxman. An earlier version of the chapter on globalization by Christine Fry was first presented as the opening keynote address at the AGHE conference in Richmond. The chapters by Kathryn (Jay) Elliott and Monica Nandan describe how cross-cultural comparison can be used to sensitize students in the United States to cultural differences in beliefs, customs, and behaviors of ethnic families and elders they are likely to serve as professionals in health care and service delivery settings. Robert Yahnke and Barbara Waxman present examples of how film (Yahnke) and literature (Waxman) can be used to teach about global aging issues. The remaining three chapters deal with issues related to aging education in Kenya, Japan, and China.

Another noteworthy feature is the diversity of disciplinary backgrounds of the authors whose work is included in this collection. The contributors come from various academic disciplines and approach the topic of global aging education in different ways. The disciplines that are represented include anthropology (Cattell, Elliott, Fry, & Ice), sociology (Gachuhi, King, Tatara and Whittington), the humanities including literature (Waxman), and film (Yahnke), social work (Nandan), gerontology (Wu), and gerontology and social welfare (Tsukada).

Christine Fry, Professor Emerita of Anthropology at Loyola University of Chicago, received her PhD in sociocultural anthropology from the University of Arizona. As one of the founding pioneers of the Association for Anthropology and Gerontology (AAGE), she was instrumental in promoting cross-cultural aging research by anthropologists. She has specialized in the anthropology of age since first living in a retirement community and then investigating the cognitive organization of the life course in the United States. Fry directed Project AGE, a cross-cultural research endeavor that examined the meaning of age and the influence of communities on the experience of aging. In her article she argues compellingly and convincingly that, although globalization is not a new phenomenon and not all bad, it threatens the wellbeing of some current and many future cohorts. Fry suggests that, to counteract this negative effect of globalization on old people, gerontologists must use their skills to work towards a moral economy that would safeguard some of the redistributive mechanisms and institutions threatened by globalization.

Kathryn (Jay) Elliott is an anthropologist whose research and teaching interests include aging among ethnic minority elders and cultural awareness in providing services to both culturally mainstream and minority elders. After completing a post-doctoral program, she worked as a researcher and clinician with Chinese elders at the University of California, San Francisco Memory Clinic and Alzheimer's Center. In her article she shows how she draws on these experiences in her teaching to provide examples from her work with Chinese elders and their families. She skillfully demonstrates the application of an anthropological approach to teaching about aging in a global context. She presents as an example her course on "Aging, Diversity, and Elder Services."

Monica Nandan received her PhD in Social Work from Florida State University. She has conducted research on various aspects of long-term care and minority aging issues. In her article, she describes the state of thanatology in U.S. college and university curricula. She presents an approach she has found useful for including cross-cultural perspectives in a course on death and dying which prepares future professionals for dealing with the multi-ethnic clientele they are likely to encounter in the practice of their professions.

Robert Yahnke is well known and respected for his work in utilizing films and literary works in teaching about aging. He has disseminated and shared this knowledge and expertise in numerous ways. He has been the Editor of the Audiovisual Review Column of *The Gerontologist* and regularly publishes both articles and book reviews that have made it possible for educators nationally to integrate the humanities more effectively into their teaching. In his chapter, Yahnke analyzes 14 international feature-length films on aging and the lifecourse in terms of three themes–of childhood and adolescence as a time of mentoring by elders, middle age as a time for resolving mid-life crises, and old age as a time for expressing wisdom and equanimity through contributions to the wider community. He presents these examples and analysis in the belief that gerontologists should have a basic understanding of the ways film communicates in the context of global aging.

Barbara Waxman is a professor of English who utilizes her expertise in literary criticism to teach students about aging. She believes that literature can change people's lives, make us more self-reflective and get us to examine our surroundings. She takes important factors like aging and gender and uses them as filters through which to view literary texts, exploring how these factors shape texts and influence readers' responses to texts. In her chapter in this volume, she uses Chilean literature in comparison to examples from the U.S. to explore views of aging in these cultural contexts and demonstrates how she utilizes this approach in teaching about aging.

Sharon King is a sociologist and research professor whose interests include caregiving and ethnicity, and aging families, religion and health. She is the first author of the paper on gerontology education and research in Kenya in which the entire session on gerontology education and research in Kenya is recounted. This includes an overview of the process that led to the Kenyatta University/Georgia State University gerontology education and research partnership. They also discuss the educational implications and cultural competence issues of gerontological research in Kenya and offer some considerations for gerontology educators and students interested in African aging. Her co-authors are Dr. Mugo Gachuhi, Coordinator of Gerontology Programs at Kenyatta University in Nairobi, Kenya; Dr. Gillian Ice in the Department of Social Medicine at the Ohio University College of Osteopathic Medicine; Dr. Maria Cattell, a Research Associate at the Field Museum of Natural History in Chicago and Dr. Frank Whittington, Director of the Gerontology Institute at Georgia State University.

Bei Wu received her PhD in gerontology from the University of Massachusetts in Boston. Before joining the faculty of Community Medicine at the West Virginia University Health Sciences Center, Dr. Wu was a Senior Research Associate at the Health Economics Research, Inc. and Center for Health Economics Research. Her main research interests are dementia and caregiving, access to care, and health service utilization among elders with chronic diseases, and minority aging. A native of China, she is bilingual and bicultural, which made her a perfect candidate for a teaching fellowship in China where she taught a course on aging policy to Chinese health care professionals. In her article, she describes the challenges and rewards of this experience and reminds us that the transfer of knowledge from one culture to another must be made thoughtfully and sensitively if it is to achieve the expected learning outcomes. Specifically, she describes the pedagogical strategies she used to make her course meaningful to non-traditional students in China.

Noriko Tsukada and Toshio Tatara give an overview of the development and current status of academic gerontology in Japan, which seems incongruous with the fact that Japan has one of the oldest populations in the world. The authors identify structural-political reasons for the slow emergence of gerontology as a field of academic study, and make recommendations for speeding up the development of academic gerontology in Japan. The authors are well qualified to speak to this matter: Dr. Tsukada holds a Master's in Gerontological Studies from Miami of Ohio and a PhD in Social Welfare from the University of California in Los Angeles where she held doctoral and post-doctoral fellowships in gerontology. She is Associate Professor at the Nihon University Graduate School of Business in Tokyo, Japan, where she teaches aging-related courses. She has conducted research on aging policy and elder abuse from a cross-cultural perspective. Her co-author, Dr. Toshio

Tatara, is in the Sociology Department at Shukutoku University in Japan.

Association for Gerontology in Higher Education (AGHE)

For those who are not familiar with the Association for Gerontology in Higher Education, AGHE is the only national membership organization devoted primarily to gerontological education. As such, it is in a unique position to develop and sponsor education and training initiatives and to involve students, educators, researchers, and officials from across the country in providing resources for older adults and for those who serve them. AGHE and its member organizations are strongly committed to the well-being of older adults. Together, AGHE and aging-studies programs in institutions of higher education strive to prepare service delivery personnel who will work directly with elderly adults; train educators who specialize in the physical and social attributes of aging; educate society at large about the processes of aging and the implications of an aging society; and instruct older adults seeking to maximize their options in a complex and challenging age. AGHE organizes an annual leadership conference for aging and higher education, produces materials that support teaching and program development in gerontology, and provides a range of services and supports for faculty and student development. Most of the papers in this special collection were originally presented at the AGHE 2004 annual leadership conference whose theme was "Global Aging." They are all published here for the first time.

Association for Anthropology and Gerontology (AAGE)

Finally, no discussion of global aging education would be complete without mentioning the Association for Anthropology and Gerontology (AAGE). AAGE was established in 1978 as a multidisciplinary group dedicated to the exploration and understanding of aging within and across the diversity of human cultures. What unites AAGE members is a perspective that is holistic, comparative, and international. In addition to anthropology, members come from a variety of academic and applied fields including the social and biological sciences, nursing, medicine, policy studies, social work, and service provision.

A useful resource for those interested in the topics discussed in this volume is *Teaching About Aging: Interdisciplinary and Cross-Cultural Perspectives* (Shenk and Sokolovsky, 1999). The teaching guide was a joint publication of AGHE and AAGE and is available for purchase from AGHE. For further information about the history and activities of AAGE, please see the Association's web site at: http://www.oucom. ohiou.edu/som/aage/.

In conclusion, we are honored to present this volume highlighting some of the numerous excellent presentations on the theme of global aging education from the AGHE conference. The AGHE leadership was clearly on targeting in identifying the important theme of global aging for this annual meeting. They provided the impetus for studying this important topic from varied multidisciplinary and interdisciplinary perspectives. We hope you will agree that the results as demonstrated here are positive and that this volume spurs on these efforts.

REFERENCE

Shenk, D., & Sokolovsky, J. (1999). *Teaching about Aging: Interdisciplinary and Cross-Cultural Perspectives*, third edition. Washington, DC: Association of Anthropology and Gerontology and the Association for Gerontology in Higher Education.

Globalization and the Experiences of Aging

Christine L. Fry, PhD

SUMMARY. Globalization is a product of urbanization and economic intensification which has escalated since the 1970s. Globalized markets have created many of the features of modern life including consumerism, increased cultural homogeneity, increased social polarization, erosion of the sovereignty of nation states, and delocalization of daily life. The consequences of globalization for older people are primarily disadvantageous. Most notably is the restructuring of the redistributive economy. The globalization of labor results in lower wages and marked social stratification. Also family life is altered with fewer relatives who must balance work and family obligations. *[Article copies available for a fee from The Haworth Document Delivery Service: 1-800-HAWORTH. E-mail address: <docdelivery@haworthpress.com> Website: <http://www.HaworthPress.com> © 2005 by The Haworth Press, Inc. All rights reserved.]*

KEYWORDS. Globalization, urbanization, capitalism, consequences for aging

Globalization and aging are phenomena that have only recently been linked. Globalization and aging go together in a very simple and demographic way. All populations are aging. This is happening at a somewhat differential rate to all nations on the globe. In the more developed

---

Christine L. Fry is Professor of Anthropology, Emerita, Loyola University Chicago, PO Box 496, Bisbee, AZ 85603 (E-mail: cfry@luc.edu).

[Haworth co-indexing entry note]: "Globalization and the Experiences of Aging." Fry, Christine L. Co-published simultaneously in *Gerontology & Geriatrics Education* (The Haworth Press, Inc.) Vol. 26, No. 1, 2005, pp. 9-22; and: *Aging Education in a Global Context* (ed: Dena Shenk, and Lisa Groger) The Haworth Press, Inc., 2005, pp. 9-22. Single or multiple copies of this article are available for a fee from The Haworth Document Delivery Service [1-800-HAWORTH, 9:00 a.m. - 5:00 p.m. (EST). E-mail address: docdelivery@haworthpress.com].

Available online at http://www.haworthpress.com/web/GGE
doi:10.1300/J021v26n01_02

nations the percentage of the total population attaining the age of 65 or greater is reaching the 13-20% mark. In less developed nations this watermark is still under 10%. Globalization and aging, however, is more complicated than demography. Globalization is an economic and political phenomenon that has and will continue to shape the life chances of all peoples around the globe.

Globalization is a part and a product of urbanization. Globalization, at the same time, is a little different in that it is a time-space compression that is a product of changes in transportation, communication, and organizational technology. In this chapter, I will look at a number of things in exploring the linkages between globalization and aging from an anthropological perspective. Specifically, I will describe the phenomena of globalization; explore the consequences of a globalized world for people of all ages; look into the lives of people whose lives have unfolded as the world became globalized; and consider and speculate a little about consequences of globalization for those who will become old in the 21st century.

GLOBALIZATION AND ANTHROPOLOGY

Globalization has taken over anthropology as the major phenomena and processes of ethnographic communities we study. This reflects the world in which we live. It is much changed from the world that we studied in the early part of the 20th century (Mintz, 1998). Urban anthropology was invented in the 1970s in response to what was happening to our traditional communities abroad and the increased need to study communities at home in the United States (Foster & Kemper, 2002). The Society for Urban Anthropology changed its name to the Society for Urban, National and Transnational/Global Anthropology in 1997 and almost immediately doubled its membership.

GLOBALIZATION AS A PROCESS

When we look at globalization two things become apparent. First, its novelty has been exaggerated. By this I mean it is a part of a long term trend in the history of our specie. Secondly, what makes it appear novel is that something quite profound has happened in the past 30 years–since 1970–which has changed the lives of many people.

As a long term trend we turn to one of the strengths of Anthropology which is to look at the big picture over an extended period of time (Adams, 1988). Our story begins some 10,000 to 12,000 years ago. At this time there were demographically only 5 million people on earth. We lived as foragers (gatherer hunters) all over the globe. There was about 1 person per 100 square miles living in social groups of about 30 people. Although people could live as long as we do today, few did. To make a long story short, sometime around 8,000 to 9,000 years ago humans began to change. Subsistence shifted toward reliance of domesticated plants and animals. With farming, the seed was sown for the modern era. The heart of this seed is that human labor became very valuable. Societies became not only interested in the amount of human labor, but in controlling the labor of others and controlling others. Following what has been identified as the agricultural revolution we see a number of changes in the way humans lived. First populations settled down into smaller territories that were exploited more intensively. Second populations started to grow. Encampments shift to a new settlement pattern associated with villages and towns. About 5,000 years ago we see the appearance of politically centralized societies we could identify as chiefdoms, and later states took their place. Towns become places of authority which then increase in size to form a city. Cities have always been outward looking–connecting the local to a larger social order. They are trade centers, political centers, and religious centers. The world became increasingly urban. The world has a number of famous cities which are amazingly old: Istanbul, Rome, Cairo, Bombay, Calcutta, Beijing, Teotihuacán, Cuzco, etc. In the 19th Century profound changes start to occur as states are transformed into nation states. These states are different from the more traditional or archaic states that preceded them. Among the distinguishing features is the fact that nation states are imagined communities with major problems of integrating very heterogeneous populations. Nation states became major building blocks of the global economy (Wallerstein, 1989). Their main role is (1) to provide for an integrated division of labor; (2) to guarantee the flow of money, goods, and people; and, (3) to facilitate economic integration.

As we get to the contemporary era, the increases in urbanization are a combined product of colonialism and maturing capitalism. Since the industrial revolution, cities have become centers of production and exchange as well as political nuclei. We have some interesting statistics concerning the recent urbanization of the globe. In 1800 only 3% of the world's population was urbanized. By 1900 the percent of the world's population that was urbanized had increased to 13% (Brum & Williams, 1983), and by 1980, the urbanized population of the world had risen to 40%. At the turn of the century (2000) 47% of the world's population is urbanized. The level of urbanization differs by economic development. In the more developed countries urbanization is at 76% while in the less developed countries only 39% of the population is urban (*http://www. un.org/popin/wdtrends.htm*, 1999).

Globalization looks like the latest stages of a 9,000-year old trend that has heated up and speeded up in the past 200 years and especially since 1970. It is the recentness of the change that makes it appear to be novel. How did we become so globalized so fast? In 1970 the post WWII prosperity faced a crisis. It is interesting to note that from 1945 to 1970 we were less global than we had been in the early 20th century. The trigger was a crisis in Fordism. This is the vision of Henry Ford that involved a combination of mass production and a unionized labor force that had the purchasing power to consume manufactured goods. This was combined with state sponsored consumerism and Keynesian fiscal management. The declining profits resulted in all the things we associate with globalization which include: off shore production; export production zones; out contracting of work; and the restructuring of the welfare state (Nash, 1989). The net result is the phenomena we identify as globalization. Most obvious are the stretching and deepening of social relations across national borders. People find that everyday activities are influenced by events that happen at great distances (Hannerz, 1992; Smith, 2001). Social scientists find that phrases such as globalized, transnational, translocal, delocalized, deterritorialized, the global village creep into our vocabulary.

Much of the technology in transportation that makes this possible is not really new. For instance, the telegraph was invented in the 19th century. The stock market has been operating on real global time since its inception. The world was divided into 24 time zones in 1880 because of railroads and the need to rationalize schedules. We do have some novel changes in social organization and technology. In the last half of the 20th century we invented supranational organizations such as the World Trade Organization, the World Bank, the United Nations, NAFTA, the European Union, and OPEC. We have devised new technologies to facilitate exchange and communication which include such things as container terminals and containerized cargo; jets–both passenger and cargo; and the internet. This all makes it possible to maintain relationships across borders.

At the root of the changes of the past 30 years are political and economic arrangements. We find borders are opened through trade agreements. Nation states alter tax laws to promote offshore production to encourage business and job creation by eliminating tariffs. Also technological improvements have resulted in inexpensive and reliable communication and transportation.

CONSEQUENCES OF GLOBALIZATION

The changes associated with globalization have consequences both good and bad. Many of these are economic, but have major consequences for the social worlds in which we live.

Availability of Consumer Goods

Consumer goods and consumerism has increased over the past 30 years. What we see crowding the aisles of Wal-Mart would not be possible if China had not entered the global economy. The reason for this is directly linked to cheap labor. Many of the products we consume such as lighting fixtures, coffee makers, irons, and computers are either stable in price or cheaper than they were 20-30 years ago. There is also more supply and availability of these products.

Increased Cultural Homogeneity

Is the world becoming increasingly homogenous? Certainly consumerism has spread. Where we see the spread of an economic form, we expect it to be followed by cultural transformation. In the colonial empire of Great Britain, it was commonly recognized that the life ways of native peoples were doomed. The main factor in the resulting cultural homogeneity is the invention of nation states, not globalization (Weber, 1976). To promote a potentially problematic integration nation states require one official language. Men also share a common experience and acculturation through military service. Universal education, in providing basic skills and knowledge about the world, results in cultural uniformity. If cultural differences are disruptive, nation states promote programs of ethnocide and genocide. On the other hand, there is evidence of a creolization of cultural forms (Garcia Canclini, 1997; Hannerz, 1992). In spite of electronic media and popular culture, much of the native cultural forms persist in modified forms at the local level.

We also have evidence of cultural resistance such as fundamentalism, Chiapas, 1968, Feminism, and ecological resistance.

Deterritorialization or Erosion of the Sovereignty of Nations

Are nation states becoming an archaic political form? Nation states in rationalizing economies face many constraints. International finance places constraints on nation states. International aid is constraining because much of it is political in nature. International trade agreements alter internal economics. Nation states also face challenges from transnational migration and from the power of transnational corporations. World migration intensified beginning around 1600, but after 1980 the very pattern is very different (Basch, Schiller, & Blanc, 1994; Kearney, 1991). Some 2% of the world's population lives and works in countries where they are not citizens and do not want to be. This translates into 100,000+ million people. The host nation welcomes the cheap labor, but not the person providing it. Transnational corporations are possibly becoming the dominant governance institution (Korton, 1995). Corporations are centered on private gain, but influence national policies. Of the top 100 global financial entities 46% are corporations; 54% are nation states. Tops in the nation state category are the United States, Japan, Germany, France, United Kingdom, Italy, China, Brazil, Canada, and Spain. A little lower in the list at 25th is General Motors, 27th Wal-Mart, 29th Exxon, and 30th Ford.

Delocalization of Ordinary Life

This is a product of urbanization and living in cities. Reference groups are no longer localized. The locale of where one lives becomes irrelevant (Durrschmidt, 1997). Often in urban environments one does not know who lives next door. Social networks are based on social factors and are no longer based on proximity.

Globalization of Production

Of all the consequences of globalization, this is the most directly economic (Rothstein & Blim, 1992). Off-shore production moves production to less developed countries. More developed economies become service economies. Production takes place in Export Production Zones where taxation on productive activities is avoided. These are production facilities that are sweat shops with laborers working for very low wages.

This arrangement places workers all over the world in direct competition with each other.

Increased Social Polarization

This refers to an increase in social stratification which perhaps is the most significant consequence of globalization. The labor force is increasingly divided into two components: the knowledge workers and the manual workers (haves and have-nots). Such labor market dualism has resulted in a declining standard of living, especially as there is a reduction of opportunities for those without education (Levine, 1995). There is even evidence that knowledge jobs are going overseas. Why pay a programmer $40-$60K a year when you can get the same work for $20K in India? This is combined with changes in welfare shifting to privatization and workfare which is resulting in depressed wages.

Increase in localization: We have some evidence for a counter trend. This is perhaps a little surprising since this goes in the opposite direction of globalization. There is evidence of increasing enclavement of people who see a disconnect with the larger world as not relevant to them. In the working class community of Momence, IL where I worked, I have had informants on their death beds tell me, "I have had a good life, a good wife, the kids are raised and that is all that counts." We have some other interesting statistics. Only 2-5% of the world's population is electronically connected–super connected, that is. These people have multiple phones and use the internet several times a day. On the other hand, 60% of the world's population has never made a phone call (Graham, 2002). There is a growing disconnection of the world's poor.

THE EXPERIENCES OF AGING IN A GLOBALIZED WORLD

What does all this have to do with real life most of which is lived at the local level? How has globalization affected real people who have grown old since 1970? I am going to give you a glimpse into the lives of a handful of people from different parts of the world–Africa, United States, and Canada. What we should see is that the effects of globalization are conditioned by where one is located in the stratification system. The higher one's social position, the more pronounced the effect of globalization.

Karui–a Herero Hunter

The Herero are a pastoral people of Southern Africa (Namibia) and Botswana. Karui was born in 1911 in Botswana. His mother was the junior wife of his father. His father fled from Namibia from the German massacre in 1904. He grew up in his father's village in Botswana. During the Second World War he was involved in the fighting, mostly digging trenches in North Africa. After the war he returned and married his first wife and set up a village with 30 cattle. His wife is his cross-cousin (mother's brother's daughter)–the marriage was arranged by his mother. He paid 2 cows and 20 pound sterling bride price. They had two boys. She returned to her family in 1953 and he did not return the bride price since he kept the children. He married his second wife in 1978–another cross cousin. Again the marriage was arranged by his mother. In this marriage, he and his wife were given two children by her relatives. He is a great hunter–some of the big things he has killed include 26 lions, 15 leopards, 9 hyenas, 11 buffalo, 30 giraffes, 27 elands, 16 gemsboks, 37 kudus, 20 wildebeests, and 6 zebras. He has been attacked by lions twice and has scars to show it. Because he is such a successful hunter, he has been the victim of witchcraft several times–cured by traditional healers. He complains that children today are disrespectful of their parents. They do not work. To make them work you have to beat them. Otherwise, they just sneak off for sex.

George–A Momence Executive

Momence is a town of a little over 3,000 located about 50 miles south of Chicago in Illinois. George was born in 1917 in Pennsylvania. He was the only child of older parents. His dad invested all he had in a hotel which burnt shortly after completion and he died soon after that. George and his mother moved in with her brother in Cleveland. Just before Pearl Harbor he got an accounting job in the aviation industry. This exempted him from service in WWII. After a couple of job changes he took a senior position in a book distributing company (in New Jersey) where he eventually became president. He was relocated to Momence, Illinois, where he bought one of the biggest houses in town and remained there ever since. This was 1964 and he was president of the entire company. Through the 1960s the company kept expanding with plants in Nevada and Georgia as well as New Jersey and Illinois. In 1971 the W. R. Grace Company bought out the book distribution company. Within a year there was conflict and George was fired. Fortunately for George, he had an employment contract and sued and won $100K per year for 15 years. He was lured out of his retirement several times to be a personnel director at a regional corporation and finally the Vice President of a local bank. He served for over 12 years as Vice President of the Momence Gladiolus Festival Association.

Florence Edenshaw Davidson–A Haida Woman

The Haida are a Native American group living on the Northwest Coast of British Columbia. The biography of Florence is recorded in *During My Time* by Margaret Blackman (1992). Florence was born in 1896 into the Raven Moiety. She is a member of the Haida Nobility. Her father was a chief. In many respects her life is very Haida. She spent her first menses in the menstrual hut. At the age of 13 she married Robert Davidson of the Eagle Moiety–he was her cross-cousin (MBS). She had 13 children–most of whom survived. By the time Florence became an adult, potlatches were outlawed by the Canadian government. Florence gave a good many very large church socials. Florence has place settings for 200 people and her living room can sit well over 100 people. Florence welcomed Queen Elizabeth and Prince Philip to the Queen Charlotte Islands–representing the Canadian government and local people. All of her children are well-connected as is she. Her father, well known artist, Charles Edensaw, carved one of the totem poles in the Field Museum in Chicago. Robert Davidson, Florence's husband, made Haida jewelry for an international art market. She celebrated her 95th birthday with a large dinner (potlatch) with 400 people in attendance.

Global events have impacts on the lives of people, regardless how isolated they are all over the world. Of the three people here our Botswana hunter is the least touched by globalization. War and the German massacre impacted him–the labor market did not. George, because of his position at the top of the corporate hierarchy and his position in the social stratification of the United States, is most globally connected. He also had to fight to get benefits. Florence is not far behind, again because she is of a high-ranked Haida family.

CONSEQUENCES OF GLOBALIZATION FOR OLDER PEOPLE

Thirty years of transformation is hardly enough time to comprehend the process much less to see how the consequences unfold in later life. Many people who grew old during this time had spent much of their adult lives when we were far less globalized. The issues most salient for people experiencing and entering old age in the present and near future are families, social stratification, and the restructuring of the welfare state.

Families

There are three issues of concern: demography, and the meaning and form of kinship. First, the Demographic Transition has altered many families. Vern Bengtson and Ariela Lowenstein (2003) in their recent book, *Global Aging and Challenges to Families* have explored the demographic consequences. There are fewer children and fewer kin in an ego's kindred. There is greater generational separation. This is Bengtson's "Bean Pole Family." With greater longevity, families are having longer shared lives at the end of the life course. There is an interesting counter trend: those who are poor continue to have large families. For them, availability of kin may not be an issue.

Secondly, the whole meaning of kinship has changed. Kinship is no longer the familiar understandings of descent and marriage implicit in the law and in most genealogies. The introduction of new reproductive technologies has radically altered our view of descent. Likewise, experimentation with alternate marriage forms other than a long term legal relationship between a man and a woman has shifted the meaning of marriage. Consequently, at the end of the 20th century descent and marriage have been replaced with a diversity of forms, and an emphasis on individualism rather than relatives (Strathern, 1992). The implication is that descent groups, as flexible as they are, may entirely evaporate. On the other hand, this may be more of a middle class issue.

Thirdly, certain forms of kinship may not be the best for people who are extremely old. The form of kinship which seems to fit with globalization is bilateral kindred with neolocal residence. Bilateral kindreds are very flexible, all-encompassing webs of relationships based on lineal (descent) and collateral (siblings–aunts/uncles) linkages. The older one becomes, the greater the chances that this network may have withered through the death of ascending relatives, many of the collaterals and, if one is unlucky, the descending connections to children.

Globalization of Labor and an Increase in Social Stratification

This should strike a sympathetic chord among gerontologists since so much of what we do in gerontology is to promote the welfare of people who have grown old and have withdrawn from the labor market or who are occupying a marginal position. Off shore production means that workers around the globe are placed in direct competition with each other. Transnational corporations with the support of nation states or local governments are able to negotiate favorable production operation and cheap labor. They also negotiate conditions that eliminate taxation. It is unclear if a sweatshop worker (usually a she) will be able to contribute much to an extended family and aging parents. Also the working life in a sweatshop is remarkably short–a female textile worker or electronics worker is old by the age of 24 or 27. This is mostly because of the demands of the work place (close work such as the detailed assembly of electronic circuits or even sewing) and associated working conditions.

Facing international competition, the standard of living for all working people has declined. With the reduction of wages, many workers find themselves working several jobs and facing a wage/time compression which makes it nearly impossible to do the work of kinship-care giving. Pensions are now deferred income. With lower wages that means less income to defer. Also with high demands in the here and now (for major consumption needs) people are likely to borrow against the future, leaving even less in the future. The real dualism in globalized labor is the divide between (1) the extremely rich who do little, but benefit from financial capitalism (investments) or own the productive organization at the international level, and (2) both the knowledge and manual workers who work for very low or relatively low wages. Life long employment (predictable and stable) is increasingly being replaced by contingency labor (short term and less predictable). We are probably just beginning to see the effects of globalization among the old as Baby Boomers are nearing retirement. With globalization of the economy, it is fairly certain that in the 21st century it will be much scarier to grow old.

Restructuring of the Welfare State

Welfare is an issue to which most gerontologists are sensitive. For instance the recent recommendation by Greenspan has sent chills down our gerontological spines. Gerontology and older people are dependent on the redistributive economy of the nation state. In the United States it is Medicare, Medicaid, Social Security, Older Americans Act, NIA, etc., that is our resource base. If the attack on these pillars continues, our foundations will get shakier. Within the past two decades we have seen challenges facing GSA as the membership base changes. The financing of globalization places constraints on nation states (International Monetary Fund or the World Bank). Consequently, we will see continued change in the redistributive economy of those states. If we look beyond the nation state into the global economy, there is no redistributive economy–there are no taxing bodies.

I think we will see storm clouds on the horizon if they are not right upon us in the here and now. It is time to start thinking about these issues to prepare ourselves for aging in a globalized world. Globalization has consequences for the life chances of everyone, not only the young who are entering the labor force, but the old who are retiring from the world of work. How can we in the multidisciplinary field of gerontology prepare for globalization? In many respects we are prepared. We have created a fairly extensive political economy of aging (Estes, 1979; Minkler & Estes, 1999). We have health care services, formalized care, income transfers and the like. AGHE is an organization working with academic programs providing advanced training for age workers. These training programs in gerontology are preparing individuals to enter the world of work in this political economy. We need to be alert to issues facing future cohorts who are experiencing the consequences of globalization more directly. Most obvious is that we are going to see more people facing old age with fewer financial resources.

The redistributive economy (taxation) is the part of the economy which supports the political economy of aging. This part of the economy is what we refer to as the moral economy–the economy that works for the good of society and its citizens. This economy is defined by nation states and the political processes which create public policies and allocate budgets. As gerontologists we need to be a part of this process to make sure the moral economy can meet the needs of its older citizens.

A globalized economy is an international political economy concerned with production, distribution and exchange for private and corporate gain. In the past 30 years we have seen tremendous expansion of this economy. At the same time we have not seen the development of a moral economy. Since most gerontological issues center on human services and human welfare, in a globalized world we should work for a moral economy that can address and respond to those issues. This means we need to impact a political economy of aging in a way that meets the needs of older adults in North America, Europe, Africa, Asia, Australia, the Pacific and South America–in short, around the globe. Who will look into the social world we have created and pay attention to the interests of older people? If we as gerontologists don't, who will?

By now it should be clear that the linkage between aging and globalization is more than demographic. In fact, without globalization, aging as we know it would be very different. The conditions that promoted the demographic transition would not have happened. Highly productive economies promoting consumerism and wage labor would not exist. People would grow old in families whose members did not face the competing demands of work and personal life. Social life would be based on proximity. Nation states would not have their sovereignty threatened by transnational corporate wealth. Moral economies promoting the welfare of citizenry would be the norm. But it did not turn out that way. Gerontology is our multidisciplinary response to work for the benefit of older people in a globalized world.

REFERENCES

Adams, R. N. (1988). *The Eighth Day: Social Evolution as the Self-Organization of Energy.* Austin: University of Texas Press.

Basch, L., Schiller, N. G., & Blanc, C. S. (1994). *Nations Unbound: Transnational Projects, Postcolonial Predicaments, and Deterritorialized Nation-State.* Amsterdam: Gordon & Breach.

Bengtson, V. L., & Lowenstein, A. (2003). *Global Aging and Challenges to Families.* New York: Springer.

Blackman, M. B. (1992). *During My Time: Florence Edenshaw Davidson, A Haida Woman.* Seattle: University of Washington Press.

Brum, S. D., & Williams, J. F. (1983). *Cities of the World: World Regional and Urban Development.* New York: Harper & Row.

Durrschmidt, J. (1997). The delinking of locale and milieu: On the situatedness of extended milieux in a global environment. In Eade, J. (Ed.), *Living in the Global City.* (pp. 56-66). London: Routledge.

Estes, C. L. (1979). *The Aging Enterprise.* San Francisco: Jossey Bass.

Foster, G. M., & Kemper, R. V. (2002). Anthropological fieldwork in cities. In Gmelch, G. & Zenner, W. P. (Eds.), *Urban Life: Readings in Urban Anthropology.* (pp. 89-101). Prospect Heights: Waveland Press.

Garcia Canclini, N. (1997). Urban cultures at the end of the century, Anthropological perspectives. *International Social Science Journal.* 153, 345-54.

Graham, S. (2002). Bridging urban digital divides? Urban polarization and information and communications technologies. *Urban Studies* 39, 33-56.

Hannerz, U. (1992) *Cultural Complexity: Studies in the Social Organization of Meaning.* New York: Columbia University Press.

Kearney, M. (1991). Borders and boundaries of state and self at the end of empire. *Journal of Historical Sociology* 4, 48-74.

Korton, D. (1995) *When Corporations Rule the World.* Hartford, CT: Kumarian Press.

Levine, M. V. (1995). Globalization and wage polarization in U. S. and Canadian cities: Does public policy make a difference? In. Kresl, P. K. & Gappart, G. (Eds.), *North American Cities and the Global Economy*. Thousand Oaks, CA: Sage.

Minkler, M., & Estes, C.L. (Eds.) (1999). *Critical Gerontology: Perspectives from Political and Moral Economy*. Amityville, NY: Baywood.

Mintz, S. (1998). The localization of anthropological practice: From area studies to transnationalism. *Critical Anthropology*. 18, 117-133.

Nash, J. (1989). *From Tank Town to High Tech*. Albany: New York Press.

Rothstein, F. A., & Blim, M. L. (Eds.) (1992) *Anthropology and the Global Factory*. New York: Bergin & Garvey.

Smith, M. P. (2001). *Transnational Urbanism*. New York: Blackwell.

Strathern, M. (1992). *After Nature: English Kinship in the Late Twentieth Century*. New York: Cambridge University Press.

United Nations Population Division (1999). *World urbanization prospects: 1999 revisions*. Retrieved February 5, 2004 from *http://www.un.org/popin/wdtrends.htm*.

Wallerstein, I. (1989). *The Modern World System III: The Second Era of Great Expansion of the Capitalist World-Economy, 1730-1840's*. New York: Academic Press.

Weber, E. (1976). *Peasants into Frenchmen: The Modernization of Rural France, 1870-1914*. Stanford: Stanford University Press.

Course Design on Aging:
Incorporating Cross-Cultural Perspectives that Challenge Assumptions About Assessment and Service Delivery

Kathryn Sabrena Elliott, PhD

SUMMARY. This article explores the benefits of using cross-cultural, anthropological approaches to help students understand the varying experience of aging within the United States and around the globe. Through cultural comparison and increased knowledge of the cultural context of aging standardized aspects of practice such as assessment protocols and concepts of function are critiqued, so that students will be better prepared to work as professionals with elders from diverse cultural backgrounds. A gerontology course designed to accomplish these goals is used as the focus of discussion and as an example of how such a course can be constructed. *[Article copies available for a fee from The Haworth Document Delivery Service: 1-800-HAWORTH. E-mail address: <docdelivery@ haworthpress.com> Website: <http://www.HaworthPress.com> © 2005 by The Haworth Press, Inc. All rights reserved.]*

KEYWORDS. Cultural diversity, elder services, cross-cultural comparison, cultural context

Kathryn Sabrena Elliott is Director, Gerontology Program and Center on Aging, Minnesota State University, Mankato, 358 Trafton Science Center N, Mankato, MN 56001 USA (E-mail: kathryn.elliott@mnsu.edu).

[Haworth co-indexing entry note]: "Course Design on Aging: Incorporating Cross-Cultural Perspectives that Challenge Assumptions About Assessment and Service Delivery." Elliott, Kathryn Sabrena. Co-published simultaneously in *Gerontology & Geriatrics Education* (The Haworth Press, Inc.) Vol. 26, No. 1, 2005, pp. 23-41; and: *Aging Education in a Global Context* (ed: Dena Shenk, and Lisa Groger) The Haworth Press, Inc., 2005, pp. 23-41. Single or multiple copies of this article are available for a fee from The Haworth Document Delivery Service [1-800-HAWORTH, 9:00 a.m. - 5:00 p.m. (EST). E-mail address: docdelivery@ haworthpress.com].

doi:10.1300/J021v26n01_03

Reconciling the need to accommodate ethnic, cultural, and other kinds of diversity with the equally important need to standardize policies, assessment protocols, best practices, and services is a major theoretical and practical challenge for gerontology. This article explores the benefits of using cross-cultural, anthropological approaches to help students understand the varying experience of aging within the U.S. and around the globe. Through cultural comparison and increased knowledge of the cultural context of aging, standardized aspects of practice are critiqued, so that students will be better prepared to work with elders from diverse cultural backgrounds. A gerontology course designed to accomplish these educational goals will be used as the focus of discussion and as an example of how such a course can be constructed.

THE IMPORTANCE OF DIVERSITY
TO BROADER GERONTOLOGICAL CONCERNS

The ethnic and cultural diversity of the United States is increasing rapidly, as is diversity within the population of American elders (Hooyman & Kiyak, 2005; Fried & Mehrotra, 1998; Gelfand, 2003; Olson, 2001). "The number of older Latinos is expected to grow by 238 percent; blacks, 134 percent; Asian Americans, 354 percent; and American Indians and Alaskan Natives, 159 percent, as compared to only 79 percent for the white, non-Latino elderly" (Olson, 2001, p. 3). Olson notes as well that many Americans are "first- and second-generation immigrants from Europe and some of these ethnic groups have particularly large and growing numbers of older people. Even those who are native born and mostly Americanized, such as the Irish, Poles, Italians, and Greeks, they retain distinctive characteristics that affect aging and long-term care" (p. 3).

Elders use disproportionately more health care and social services than younger age groups (Hooyman & Kiyak, 2005; Moody, 2002). Increasing need for services associated with aging is bringing more and more culturally diverse elders into clinical and social service settings in which their worldviews, values and behaviors are very different from those of "the middle-class, White, Christian, nonimmigrant . . . practitioner" (Fried & Mehrotra, 1998, p. xv). These cross-cultural encounters can be fraught with misunderstanding and loss of opportunity unless service providers have "culturally relevant . . . competencies essential for designing, implementing, and evaluating effective programs for a diverse array of older adults" (p. xvi).

The increasing cultural and ethnic diversity of the American population has highlighted the need to apply anthropological knowledge to the delivery of human services in general (Green, 1999) and to healthcare and clinical services specifically (Shimkin & Golde, 1983; Rush, 1996). It has also resulted in the development of ethnogerontology as a growing sub-field within social gerontology (Hooyman & Kiyak 2005; Stoller & Gibson, 2000). Gelfand (1994, 2003) and Yee (2002) link ethnic diversity explicitly with its implications for elder services, exemplifying the shift in ethnogerontology from awareness of cultural differences to discussion of the kind of knowledge and skills needed to be culturally competent.

The cumulative knowledge of anthropologists who have studied aging cross-culturally is crucial to understanding the sociocultural dimension in human aging and its many possible variations. This knowledge can be applied to the delivery of services to culturally diverse elders, inside and outside of the United States (Holmes & Holmes, 1995; Keith et al., 1994; Sokolovsky, 1997). Comparing different cultures allows us to understand that there are areas of shared human concern as people face existential challenges that are universal. It also makes us aware that different cultures can respond in strikingly different ways to the same challenges. Comparison of this kind enhances understanding of our own culture, as well as other cultures. Understanding particular aspects of a culture in the context of the whole helps outsiders understand the meaning of these particulars for the "natives" of that culture. Such understanding cannot be achieved "when facts are taken out of context, and there has been a long history of faulty thinking that has resulted from this practice" (Holmes & Holmes, 1995, p. 9).

Cross-Cultural Comparison and Cultural Context as Didactic Strategies

Cross-cultural comparison and an in-depth, nuanced and holistic understanding of cultural context are analytical approaches drawn from the classic disciplinary perspective of anthropology. They have both proven to be powerful didactic strategies in the course described here. They constitute the backbone onto which the course has been built and are employed from the very first day of the semester, on which the film "Postville: When Cultures Collide" (Iowa Public Television, 2001) is shown about a town in Iowa of 1500 people that is suddenly transformed economically and culturally by the arrival of 300 Hasidic Jews. The newcomers open a kosher meat processing plant and then hire Mexican immigrants to work in it, adding another 400 people to the town's population. This film introduces students right away to the issues of culture, cultural clashes, and cross-cultural communication that will reverberate throughout the entire semester in other films and in readings, written assignments, discussions, and class exercises. Cross-cultural comparison and emphasis on understanding cultural context allow the course to expand progressively outward in scope as it explores cultural differences and their relevance for aging and elder services, moving eventually from considering a small town in Iowa at the beginning of the course to examining the impact on elders of the political economies of entire nation-states in global context by the end of the semester.

Topics in Gerontology Course: "Aging, Diversity, and Elder Services"

This course was originally designed as a graduate seminar in gerontology and taught twice in that format. It was then revised and taught twice more as a class that was taken by both upper-level undergraduates and graduate students. The graduate students who have taken this course thus far include masters' candidates in gerontology, as well as graduate students from communication disorders, health science, and nursing. Undergraduates in the class have included majors in social work, nursing and ethnic studies. Most of these students intended to pursue careers in which they would be providing services to and working directly with elders and their families.

Common knowledge shared by the students included an awareness that the American population is becoming increasingly more diverse culturally and that this is true even in a state like Minnesota, which has a predominantly white population that is ethnically European in background, something reflected in the predominantly white population of Minnesotans currently sixty-five and older (Holmquist, 1981; Minnesota Board on Aging, 1998a, p. 8). Students had received first-hand experience interacting with individuals from growing Hispanic, Somali, and Hmong communities in Minnesota consistent with the increasing cultural diversity of elders in the state (Minnesota Board on Aging, 1998b, 1998c). Students expected to be working with clients/patients and families from diverse cultural backgrounds at some point in their future careers and came to the class with a desire to learn not only about cultural and ethnic differences in general within the U.S. and cross-na-

tionally but also about the practical relevance these differences would–
and should–have in their future professional work. Thus, to meet both
the needs of these students and of the diverse elders and families with
whom they would very likely work, this course was designed with the
core didactic task of connecting cultural/ethnic diversity with its implications for the design and delivery of elder services.

Course Objectives: Imparting the Knowledge and Skills of Cultural Competence

Emphasis in training service providers to meet the needs of diverse
elders has shifted from "cultural sensitivity (awareness of cultural differences)" to cultural competence, which Hooyman and Kiyak define as
"specific knowledge and skills to work effectively with ethnic minorities" (2005, p. 554). Many healthcare providers, in particular, recognize
the importance of incorporating cross-cultural knowledge into the delivery of services and have developed models for effective cross-cultural practice. One such example is the model for culturally responsive
healthcare developed by Vawter, Culhane-Pera, Babbitt, Xiong, and
Solberg (2003) working with the Hmong community in Minnesota.
Vawter et al.'s model incorporates the kind of knowledge and many of
the skills that are included in the learning objectives of the gerontology
course described here. There are seven learning objectives, which, as a
whole, are intended to combine mastery of certain types of knowledge
with skills involved in applying that knowledge to practice and service
delivery (2003).

CULTURAL DIVERSITY CORE PRINCIPLES TO IMPART TO FUTURE PRACTITIONERS

The course instructor worked for three years as a medical anthropologist and ethnogerontologist in an Alzheimer's research project involv-
ing the Chinese community in San Francisco. Serving as a member of
the clinical team at an Alzheimer's clinic, she collected and analyzed
data on the sociocultural factors influencing the medical evaluation,
case management and family care of demented Chinese elders and their
use of health and social support services. She conducted family interviews as a part of patient medical evaluations, participated in diagnostic
case and family conferences and helped conceptualize care plans in a
culturally responsive way for Chinese patients and their families. In ad-

dition, she helped develop and test Alzheimer's education outreach strategies targeted at San Francisco's Chinese community (Elliott & Di Minno, in press; Elliott, Di Minno, Lam & Tu, 1996). Drawing on her own applied experience and from the literature in applied and medical anthropology, ethnogeriatrics, and ethnogerontology (Green, 1999; Helman, 2001; Loustaunau & Sobo, 1997; Yeo & Gallagher-Thompson, 1996; Valle, 1998), she identified six core principles as ones that are particularly important for students to understand if they are to apply knowledge of cultural/ethnic diversity effectively to practice "on the front lines" with elders. Because elders are members of families and of communities, the course emphasizes that working effectively with the social groups that shape the daily lives of elders is crucial for successfully providing services. The course structure, materials and assignments are designed to reinforce these core principles in combination with the learning objectives.

1. *Culture is flexible, constantly changing, dynamic and complex.* There are contradictory and/or competing values and social patterns within any given culture that are responded to in different ways by different families and by different individuals within the same family or other social group.
2. *There is much diversity within any given cultural or ethnic group.* This is true not only at the individual and family level, but also with regard to sub-groups within broad categories. Such differences include immigration history (when, how, and why this particular elder and the elder's family immigrated to the United States); specific region within a homeland from which elders and their families may have emigrated; language/dialect spoken; and tribal group (as in the case of Native Americans and immigrants from Africa).
3. *General cultural knowledge about the shared values, kinship system, religion, health-related beliefs and practices, etc., of any given ethnic or cultural group must not be stereotyped.* Practitioners need to learn the general body of cultural knowledge related to specific ethnic/cultural groups, as one would learn any generalized body of knowledge about, for example, the physiology of aging bodies or the array of elder services available in a given community. Practitioners should then apply this knowledge on a case-by-case basis, much as they would other generalized bodies of knowledge. What is or is not true about–or relevant for–this particular elder and his/her family?

4. *The cultural and social context of any human being's life has a tremendous influence on that human being's worldview and on the way in which a person navigates through life and relates to others in his/her social group.* Anthropological research has firmly established that the definition of "family" varies across cultural settings. This is also true of beliefs about who is the most appropriate caregiver for a frail elder. Individuals seek assistance from others in their social environment in ways that are culturally patterned. Cultural beliefs not only influence whether or not individuals decide that they are ill, but also their identification of the illness as a specific one with a specific cause, course of treatment and prognosis. Guided by what medical anthropologists have termed culturally patterned "hierarchies of resort" sick individuals and their families decide what kind of healer(s) can cure that particular illness, what other treatments are available for it and which should be options of first or last resort (Brown, 1998, p. 45). Cultural and social context also influences who will make medical decisions for a sick individual. (The oldest son, as the designated family decision maker in a traditionally oriented Chinese family, for example, is the one with the culturally sanctioned authority to make medical decisions for an incapacitated family elder.) If service providers are unaware of the worldviews shaping client expectations about eldercare and assistance with health problems, the resulting cultural clash may create barriers to service delivery by increasing misunderstanding or even provoking outright rejection of services that could otherwise have been adapted in a culturally acceptable way.

5. *We all come from specific cultural/ethnic backgrounds and have culturally shaped beliefs, practices, kinship relationships, moral attitudes and worldviews.* This is as true for clinicians and service providers as it is for any other human beings. The unconscious assumptions health and social service providers routinely make in their lives, and in their practice, about: "normal," "rational," "functional/dysfunctional" behavior for elders and others within a family; what the explanation is for an elder's illness; whether or not Western biomedicine is effective in curing illnesses, etc., are rooted in their own cultural backgrounds. These cultural assumptions are very often not shared by people from cultural backgrounds that are strikingly different from that of the service provider. The risk for serious cultural clashes to occur in this situation is very great. Achieving a successful service or clinical out-

come is a matter of understanding both the cultural/ethnic background of an elder and the potential difficulties created in a clinical/service encounter by our own cultural assumptions.

6. *To understand ethnic minority and other culturally diverse elders and serve them effectively, service providers must enter into the cultural and social world of the particular elder they are trying to help.* This means listening carefully to the stories elders and families from cultural backgrounds different from that of the service provider tell during service/clinical encounters about their lives, beliefs and values. Valle (1998), Green (1999) and Elliott et al. (1996) emphasize the need to enlist bicultural, bilingual service providers and forge links with trusted leaders and organizations within a community. It is important to learn about both the cultural beliefs and practices of particular ethnic/cultural groups and how they do–or do not–play out in the specific, local community to which services are being offered. Most importantly, service providers must learn to respect and work with–and within–a given cultural world in order to provide effective care.

COURSE MATERIALS AND ASSIGNMENTS

In the most recent incarnation of this course, two main text books were required: *Age Through Ethnic Lenses: Caring for the Elderly in a Multicultural Society*, edited by Laura Katz Olson (2001) and Donald Gelfand's *Aging and Ethnicity: Knowledge and Services* (1994), which has recently come out in a second edition (2003). Katz's book includes chapters that specifically profile an array of ethnic/cultural and other forms of diversity relevant to the aging experience, including their implications for elder-services. Gelfand's book provides specific information about diverse groups and explicitly addresses the implications of diversity for the design and delivery of elder services. Selected additional readings were put on reserve in the library. The *Journal of Cross-Cultural Gerontology* has been a particularly valuable source of such additional readings.

Assignments included two take-home essay exams in which students must think with the facts in a creative and applied way and a research paper requiring students to research a topic of their choice related to diversity and aging, explicitly addressing already existing models of service design for diverse elders or the applied implications of their paper topic for the structure and delivery of such services. A number of in-class exercises have also been created for students to work on as a group. The viewing and in-depth class discussion of a variety of films is integral to this course. Films have been chosen to illustrate important aspects of diversity, with particular emphasis placed on enriching students' understanding of the cultural context of diverse aging experiences. This encourages them to reflect on their own culture and use cross-cultural comparison to critique the cultural assumptions embedded in standardized gerontological concepts and assessments.

Basic Structure of the Course

The following class topics are distributed across the fourteen weeks as follows: (1) Introduction to course; (2) The Importance of Diversity to Broader Gerontological Concerns; Ethnicity and Aging in the United States; (3) Caregiving, Family, and Social Support Networks; East and Southeast Asian Elders; (4) Latino Americans; (5) African Americans; (6) Native Americans; (7) Cultural Variations on a European Background; (8) Socioreligious Groups; Death and Dying; Rural Aging; (9) Gender and Sexual Orientation; Physical and Financial Security; (10) The Implications of Diversity for Elder Services; Health, Diversity, and Elder Services; (11) Health, Diversity, and Elder Services continued; (12) Political Economy, Age, and Elder Services Across Cultures; (13) Age, Health, and Functionality Across Cultures; (14) What we can learn from studying aging and diversity in our own society and across cultures that can improve gerontological practice and service delivery for all elders. Limited space here precludes a detailed discussion of how each of these topics is approached in the course, but selected topics will be discussed.

ETHNICITY AND AGING IN THE UNITED STATES

Stanford and Yee (1991) have criticized comparisons "of blacks to whites relative to health status and access to healthcare" as implying "that minorities need to 'catch up' to whites." Such comparisons "suffer from an effort to draw conclusions about 'minority' populations, because" they "are grounded in an assumption of a 'majority' standard (for level of education, savings needed to maintain lifestyle in retirement, willingness to provide intergenerational caregiving, etc.)." An alternative approach is to acquire knowledge "in the context of the experiences and behavior of discrete population groups" (p. 12). "Focusing on the diversity within target populations–on the 'traditional' and also on the 'Americanized' versions of cultural values that determine whether events are defined as problems or challenges, social burdens or role responsibilities–can provide new energy and perspectives." These, in turn, contribute to "our definition of problems, and . . . our development of solutions" (p. 14).

The diversity and aging course described here takes the alternate approach recommended by Stanford and Yee to ethnicity in the United States. Olson's point, cited above, about the cultural diversity that exists among Americans of European descendant makes it clear that this approach is relevant to whites as well as members of ethnic minorities. Understanding aging within the context of specific populations is also a powerful approach to other types of diversity addressed in this course, such as aging in rural and in gay/lesbian communities.

Ethnicity involves a shared sense of peoplehood rooted in a distinctive sociocultural heritage, social support systems and social status. It serves as "an integrating force" for individuals as they pass "through significant life changes and transitions," "a buffer to stresses of old age" and "a filter to the aging process, influencing beliefs, behaviors, and interactions with formal and informal supports" (Hooyman & Kiyak, 2005, p. 526). The first three chapters assigned in Gelfand (1994, 2003) emphasize the multiple dimensions of ethnicity, its complexity and shifting nature and its relationship to social identity. He also addresses the positive and negative aspects of ethnicity with regard to aging and service use. Students are asked to start thinking about the strengths of diverse individuals, families and communities, "the varied coping mechanisms that grow out of different traditions" and how it might be possible "to mobilize them in service to older adults" (Fried & Mehrotra, 1998, p. xvii).

The distinction between ethnicity and ethnic minority status is emphasized. Ethnic minority groups have less power vis-à-vis the dominant group or groups in society. They face discrimination and "perceive themselves as being the objects of discrimination because of their inferior position" (Gelfand, 2003, p. 7). This discrimination can lead to legal, economic, social and subjective deprivation (p. 7). Hooyman and Kiyak's discussion of cultural, economic, and structural barriers to service utilization is introduced at this point (2005, pp. 554-558). These barriers include cultural isolation, language differences, limited access to public benefits, real or perceived discrimination by service providers and geographic distance from services.

This class session also introduces the five major ethnic/racial categories used by the U.S. Federal Government and frequently by researchers as well: White, Asian/Pacific Islander, Hispanic American, African American and American Indian. Despite problems associated with comparing all other ethnic groups against whites, contrasting data on the last four categories, which are officially designated as "ethnic minorities," to data on whites has yielded important insight into the comparative deprivation suffered by ethnic minorities and its impact on the health and economic status of ethnic minority elders (Stoller & Gibson, 2000; Johnson & Smith, 2002). Nonetheless, all five of these categories conceal much intra-group diversity, making them of limited value in designing and delivering services to specific populations. The Asian/Pacific Islander category alone, for example, encompasses a huge portion of the earth's surface and the many, very different cultural groups that inhabit it. It is emphasized to students that this category tells us nothing about the distinct languages, histories, religions, and cultures of immigrants from Pakistan, China, Cambodia, and Samoa and their practical relevance for assessing needs and delivering services to individuals from these diverse backgrounds.

After the basic parameters of ethnicity are laid out in relationship to service delivery, students are invited to identify and discuss their own ethnicity. This brings home to the students that they themselves come from a particular cultural background. Most of the students in this class thus far have a European ethnic background and are from Minnesota or the upper Midwest. They demonstrated detailed knowledge about immigrant experiences of grandparents and great-grandparents and cultural beliefs and practices passed down in their families that is consistent with scholarly work done on these groups (Conzen, 2003; Holmquist, 1981; Gjerde & Qualey, 2002; Anderson & Blanck, 2001). Ethnic self-identification led to lively discussions about the varying ethnic backgrounds of students, the cultural relevance of these and whether these cultural/ethnic backgrounds had current relevance in their own lives. Because they had already been introduced to the concept of identifying barriers to service use within a cultural/ethnic community, as well as community strengths that enhance service delivery, students were encouraged to consider whether or not their ethnicity has influenced their own use of services.

CAREGIVING, FAMILY AND SOCIAL SUPPORT NETWORKS

The family is "the primary source of social support for older adults" (Hooyman & Kiyak, 2005, p. 307). Because family is a universal institution, it is an area of shared concern among human beings (Holmes &

Holmes, 1995, p. 111). Cross-cultural empathy and communication between service providers and recipients can be built upon this common concern. However, service providers must understand that "families exist in an almost unbelievable variety of forms" (p. 111). This variety includes forms that can violate the service provider's own deeply held cultural beliefs about what a family is, who is a family member and who is not, how one can become a family member, who makes decisions for the family, the status of elderly members within it and who is the culturally designated family caregiver for a frail elder. Providers must enter and work within the world of diverse elders and families they are trying to help by understanding how profoundly different these variables can be and how emotionally and morally committed human beings are to the values and structure of the "family" associated with their own cultural definition of it.

The kinds of social support, informal care, or formal services available to elders in need of assistance can be restricted or expanded according to how rigid or permeable the boundary is between who is defined as "family" and who is not. Some kinship structures have permeable boundaries with social mechanisms to recruit "fictive kin," who then take on many of the responsibilities of a "real" family member, including eldercare. For example, McBride and Parreno (1996) describe the traditional Filipino family as "an open system, absorbing new members not only by marriage but also through kinship, compassionate friendships, or feelings of indebtedness" (p. 126). They give the example of a 24-year-old Filipino-American woman who, as "a member of the household . . . was asked to be the companion to a frail 83-year-old family friend. She was expected to take this role three times a week, while going to graduate school, juggling two part-time jobs, and maintaining her outside interests." At the same time, preparations were being made "to incorporate the elder into the family household" (p. 129). In a number of African-American communities, "local church congregations . . . are predominantly female and consist of groups of blood relatives" (Lewis & Ausberry, 1996, p. 169). This "church family" is "a natural support group that can and does respond to the many needs of African American frail elders" and within which "young parishioners are expected to care for elders with mental and physical needs" (p. 169). Mechanisms for recruiting "fictive kin" also exist in Latino communities, including *compadrazgo,* a network of kinlike ties among very close friends who exchange tangible assistance and social support" (Stoller & Gibson, 2000, p. 207).

Flexibly defined "families" like this contrast sharply with tradition-ally structured Chinese families in which the wife of the eldest son is the specifically designated primary caregiver for her parents-in-law and a clear distinction is made between who is a family member and who is not. For Chinese-American families which still adhere to the traditional Chinese definition of the family, "it is inappropriate for daughters" who have married out of the family in which they were born to "intervene in what is now someone else's family" with regard to the care of their own elderly parents (Elliott et al., 1996, p. 95). A service provider must be aware of the structures and values that influence family decisions about eldercare and whether or not "fictive kin" can be recruited to assist with it. This knowledge can help providers map the kin and "fictive kin" available to a frail elder in a way that accurately reflects the capacity of diverse families to provide eldercare and to recruit additional caregivers if necessary. When service providers can assess eldercare needs in rela-tionship to varying definitions of "family," they increase their ability to identify eldercare needs that remain unmet and why they are not being met. This may be due to rigid boundaries that limit recruitment of addi-tional family caregivers, to lack of economic resources in an extended family group that would otherwise provide care or to definitions of the family that may themselves be changing under the pressure of immigra-tion. A practitioner who understands the kinds of care that families are good–or not very good–at providing and why, will have a better sense of how formal services might be combined with family care.

Ang Lee's film "Pushing Hands" (Hope, Schamus, Liu & Lee, 1991) has been particularly effective in bringing home to students how differ-ent intergenerational relationships and family caregiving obligations to-wards elders can be from one culture to another. The film also facilitates a transition at this point in the course from the introduction of concepts relevant to diversity and service provision to an examination of how these concepts can be applied within varied sociocultural contexts. In "Pushing Hands" a Chinese elder emigrates from the People's Republic of China to join his son, his white American daughter-in-law and young grandson in the New York metropolitan area. The clash of cultural ex-pectations between this elder and his daughter-in-law and the gradual evolution of both characters towards understanding the cultural per-spective of each other drives the plot and has inspired class discussions in which students spoke with real passion about the family loyalties and cultural contradictions portrayed in this film. The elder's response to these clashes and the decision he ultimately makes to live alone in his own apartment in New York's Chinatown also realistically echo the experience of many immigrant Chinese elders who choose a living arrangement that is not traditional in order to embed themselves in an ethnic enclave that will support continued participation in the culture of their homeland. The course instructor encountered Chinese elders in her own work in San Francisco who had made the same difficult choice and she shares these real-life examples with students during class discussion of the film.

This film draws its viewers into the social and cultural world of an elderly Chinese immigrant. It addresses the feelings and beliefs surrounding "family" of all its main characters and portrays everyone's struggle to resolve conflicts over this elder's living arrangements and need for social integration. Resolution is achieved through compromises the characters make and also by drawing upon culturally appropriate resources available outside the family. The film reinforces the sixth core diversity principle described above by illustrating how important it is to enter the sociocultural world of elders and their families. Doing this helps providers understand what individuals believe and why, how beliefs can motivate behavior and how individuals, including elders, may cope with the challenges of old age in a way that is not traditional by turning to extra-familial options and resources. This knowledge can help providers design elder services and offer them in venues that are culturally appropriate and increase the chance that they will be utilized. In both "Pushing Hands" and the course instructor's research in San Francisco, it is the combination of senior housing independent of family, a non-traditional arrangement, and its location within the ethnic enclave of Chinatown that makes this option acceptable.

EAST AND SOUTHEAST ASIAN ELDERS; LATINO AMERICANS; AFRICAN AMERICANS; NATIVE AMERICANS; CULTURAL VARIATIONS ON A EUROPEAN BACKGROUND

In this section the course explores the relationship among diversity, aging and elder services within major ethnic categories and specific cultural/ethnic communities, reinforcing both the core diversity principles and the learning objectives. Students learn about the cultural characteristics of specific ethnic groups they are likely to encounter in their own professional work, such as Hmong, Somali, and Latinos. In class exercises they also practice assessing the strengths of diverse communities, identifying service barriers and incorporating this knowledge into proposals for service design and delivery. Students have the opportunity to compare diverse groups with each other and with their own cultural backgrounds. The variability within each major ethnic category that has been emphasized earlier is illustrated with specific, service-relevant examples. One such example is the cautionary reminder that the well-documented importance of Christian churches in many African-American communities as sources of social and economic support cannot be extended to Somali communities, which are Muslim. Instead we need to ask what role mosques and other organizations indigenous to these communities play.

The impact on elders of ethnic minority status and the legal, economic, and social deprivation that accompany life-long discrimination are also examined through specific examples in this section of the course. Hooyman and Kiyak (2005) emphasize that two "distinct issues should be kept in mind" with regard to ethnic minority elders: (1) "the unique historical and cultural calendar of life events and their impact on aging, many of which are positive and sources of strength and resilience"; and (2) "the consequences of racism, ageism, discrimination, and prolonged poverty, most of which are negative and perpetuate inequities across the life span" (p. 528). Cultural beliefs and behaviors should not be confused with deprivation associated with ethnic minority status. For example, when an impoverished elder eats high fat foods, this may be because he cannot afford healthier foods rather than the result of dietary preferences that are culturally shaped. The film "To Be Old, Black, and Poor" (Films for the Humanities & Sciences, Inc., 1993) has been particularly effective in communicating these distinctions to students with regard to African Americans. In this film, an impoverished African-American elder tries to care for his disabled wife, scavenging food and barricading their apartment against break-ins in a high-crime neighborhood. A variety of service providers attempt to help, but suffer from lack of coordination and sometimes work directly against each other. The situation portrayed is quite sobering for students, both with regard to the impact of poverty and crime on this elderly couple and to the contradictions within the service delivery system available to them.

THE IMPLICATIONS OF DIVERSITY FOR ELDER SERVICES

In this class meeting, students pull together and summarize what they have learned thus far about diversity in relationship to elder services. The class begins with a learning exercise on thinking about "security" and service provision to elders from multiple perspectives, keyed to a chapter on security in Gelfand in which he explores the different meanings of "security"–physical, financial, health, and personal. The exercise asks students to stop and think about the different meanings "security" can have in varying sociocultural contexts and how a consideration of these meanings and contexts will influence one's ideas about the kind of "security" services one might conceivably offer to diverse elders and their families. Seen in this light, not having to fear homophobic attacks certainly contributes to "security" for older gay men, lesbians and bisexuals, as does freedom from a long-term care "environment that is insensitive, antagonistic, and discriminatory toward them and their needs" (Claes & Moore, 2001, p. 218). The example used in this exercise of retiring FBI agents preparing for second careers is based on an actual encounter the course instructor had with a soon-to-be-retired FBI agent who was exploring the possibility of starting a business with some of his colleagues that would provide "security" services to elders, but who initially saw "security" only in law enforcement terms.

In this exercise the instructor plays the role of one of the FBI agents, who has hired the consultants, grilling the class on exactly what they mean by some of their recommendations and how the agents should actually go about building up their business and approaching prospective clients. Students usually become engrossed in this exercise and express afterwards to the instructor that they have enjoyed it. It also stimulates lively discussion about using the knowledge and skills of cultural competence that they have already had the opportunity to practice in the course. At this point the instructor emphasizes that applying cultural knowledge to service delivery is not as straightforward as it may appear at times, demonstrating this with an example from Henderson, Gutierrez-Mayka, Garcia, and Boyd (1993) about developing Alzheimer's support groups in an African-American community. Henderson et al.'s unexpected adventure in the application of cultural knowledge to service delivery reminds students that being aware of what is culturally important and service relevant within a particular cultural or ethnic group is not enough. They must know how these cultural features and the loyalties associated with them play out in particular local contexts in order to apply this knowledge effectively.

OUTCOMES AND CONCLUSION

On the last day students summarize and share with the class what they feel they have learned in the course. They also give oral presentations on their research papers, explaining in detail how they have connected cultural knowledge with its application to service design and delivery. Then, as a group, they summarize what they think gerontology as a whole can learn from studying aging in diverse contexts and across cultures. They are asked to give specific examples about how they think these new insights might contribute to gerontology's "definition of problems, and . . . development of solutions" (Stanford & Yee, 1993, p. 14).

The course has been revised several times since its inception based on oral and written feedback from students. In this feedback, they identified the following as particularly effective in helping them to meet the learning objectives: specific examples of applying knowledge to service delivery drawn from the instructor's own experience and from readings and films; opportunities to apply knowledge and skills, such as assessing community strengths and barriers to service, in class exercises; and the use of films to draw students into cultural worlds different from their own. In the student evaluations of the latest incarnation of the course, the one described in this article, cumulative scores rating 15 course elements ranged from 4.00 to 4.86, out of a total of 5. Among these scores were the following: quality of questions or problems raised by the instructor (4.43); answers to student questions (4.43); the course as a whole (4.71); amount you learned in the course (4.71); evaluative and grading techniques (4.71); and course organization (4.71). Past students have also emailed the instructor describing how what they learned helped them present on diversity issues in other gerontology courses. In looking over course materials, one of the students "realized what a wealth of material is included. . . . Thank you. I really learned a lot."

REFERENCES

Anderson, P. J. & Blanck, D. (Eds.). (2001). *Swedes in the Twin Cities: Immigrant life and Minnesota's urban frontier.* St. Paul, MN: Minnesota Historical Society Press.

Brown, P. J. (Ed.). (1998). *Understanding and applying medical anthropology.* Mountain View, CA: Mayfield Publishing Company.

Claes, J. A., & Moore, W. R. (2001). Caring for gay and lesbian elderly. In L. K. Olson (Ed.), *Age through ethnic lenses: Caring for the elderly in a multicultural society.* Lanham, MD: Rowman & Littlefield.

Conzen, K. N. (2003). *Germans in Minnesota.* St. Paul, MN: Minnesota Historical Society P ress.

Elliott, K. S., & Di Minno, M. (in press). Unruly grandmothers, ghosts and ancestors: Chinese elders and the importance of culture in dementia evaluations. *Journal of Cross-Cultural Gerontology.*

Elliott, K. S., Di Minno, M., Lam, D., & Tu, A. M. (1996). Working with Chinese families in the context of dementia. In G. Yeo & D. Gallagher-Thompson (Eds.), *Ethnicity & the dementias* (pp. 89-108). Washington, DC: Taylor & Francis.

Films for the Humanities & Sciences, Inc. (Producer). (1993). *To be old, black, and poor* [Film]. (Available from Films for the Humanities & Sciences, Inc., P.O. Box 2053, Princeton, NJ 08543-2053)

Fried, S. B., & Mehrotra, C. M. (1998). *Aging and diversity: An active learning experience.* Washington, DC: Taylor & Francis.

Gelfand, D. E. (1994). *Aging and ethnicity: Knowledge and services.* New York: Springer Publishing Company.

Gelfand, D. E. (2003). *Aging and ethnicity: Knowledge and services* (2nd ed.). New York: Springer Publishing Company.

Gjerde, J., & Qualey, C. C. (2002). *Norwegians in Minnesota.* St. Paul, MN: Minnesota Historical Society Press.

Green, J. W. (1999). *Cultural awareness in the human services: A multi-ethnic approach.* Boston: Allyn and Bacon.

Helman, C.G. (2001). *Culture, health and illness* (4th ed.). London: Arnold.

Henderson, J. N., Gutierrez-Mayka, M., Garcia, J., & Boyd, S. (1993). A model for Alzheimer's disease support group development in African-American and Hispanic populations. *The Gerontologist* 33: 409-414.

Holmes, E. R., & Holmes, L. D. (1995). *Other cultures, elder years* (2nd ed.). Thousand Oaks, CA: Sage Publications.

Holmquist, J. D. (Ed.). (1981). *They chose Minnesota: A survey of the state's ethnic groups.* St. Paul, MN: Minnesota Historical Society Press.

Hooyman, N. R., & Kiyak, H. A. (2005). *Social gerontology: A multidisciplinary perspective,* 6th edition. Boston: Allyn and Bacon.

Hope, T., Schamus, J., Liu, E., & Lee, A. (Producers), & Lee, A. (Director). (1991). *Pushing Hands* [Film]. (Available from Triboro Entertainment Group).

Iowa Public Television (Producer). (2001). *Postville: When cultures collide* [Film]. (Available from PBS Video).

Johnson, J. C., & Smith, N. H. (2002). Health and social issues associated with racial, ethnic, and cultural disparities: Differences in access and quality of care. *Generations 26*; 25-32.

Keith, J., Fry, C. L., Glascock, A. P., Ikels, C., Dickerson-Putman, J., Harpending, H. C., & Draper, P. (1994). *The aging experience: Diversity and commonality across cultures.* Thousand Oaks, CA: Sage.

Lewis, I. D., & Ausberry, M. S. C. (1996). African American families: Management of demented elders. In G. Yeo & D. Gallagher-Thompson (Eds.), *Ethnicity & the dementias* (pp. 167-174). Washington, DC: Taylor & Francis.

Loustaunau, M. O., & Sobo, E. J. (1997). *The cultural context of health, illness, and medicine.* Westport, CT: Bergin & Garvey.

McBride, M. R., & Parreno, H. (1996). Filipino American families and caregiving. In G. Yeo & D. Gallagher-Thompson (Eds.), *Ethnicity & the dementias* (pp. 123-135). Washington, DC: Taylor & Francis.

Minnesota Board on Aging. (1998a). *Aging Initiative: Project 2030: Briefing book.* St. Paul, MN: Minnesota Department of Human Services.

Minnesota Board on Aging. (1998b). *Aging Initiative: Project 2030: Policy report: Preparing for the future: Minnesotans identify opportunities and challenges for an aging society.* St. Paul, MN: Minnesota Department of Human Services.

Minnesota Board on Aging. (1998c). *Aging Initiative: Project 2030: Data report: Population profiles: African American elders, American Indian elders, Asian American elders, Hispanic elders.* St. Paul, MN: Minnesota Department of Human Services.

Moody, H. R. (2002). *Aging: Concepts and controversies* (4th ed.). Thousand Oaks, CA: Pine Forge Press.

Olson, L. K. (Ed.). (2001). *Age through ethnic lenses: Caring for the elderly in a multicultural society.* Lanham, MD: Rowman & Littlefield.

Rush, J. A. (1996). *Clinical anthropology: An application of anthropological concepts within clinical settings.* Westport, CT: Praeger.

Shimkin, D. B. & Golde, P. (Eds.). (1983). *Clinical anthropology: A new approach to American health problems?* Lanham, MD: University Press of America.

Sokolovsky, J. (Ed.). (1997). *The cultural context of aging: Worldwide perspectives* (2nd ed.). Westport, CT: Bergin & Garvey.

Stanford, E. P. & Yee, D. L. (1991). Gerontology and the relevance of diversity. *Generations 15: Diversity, new approaches to ethnic minority aging:* 11-14.

Stoller, E. P. & Gibson, R. C. (Eds.). (2000). *Worlds of difference: Inequality in the aging experience* (3rd ed.). Thousand Oaks, CA: Pine Forge Press.

Thirteen/WNET & BBC-TV (Producers). (1993). *Medicine at the crossroads: Life support* [Film]. (Available from PBS Video)

Valle, R. (1998). *Caregiving across cultures: Working with dementing illness and ethnically diverse populations.* Washington, DC: Taylor & Francis.

Vawter, D. E., Culhane-Pera, K. A., Babbitt, B., Xiong, P. & Solberg, M. M. (2003). A model for culturally responsive health care. In K.A. Culhane-Pera, D. E. Vawter, P. Xiong, B. Babbitt & M. M. Solberg (Eds.), *Healing by heart: Clinical and ethical case stories of Hmong families and Western providers* (pp. 297-342). Nashville, TN: Vanderbilt University Press.

Yee, D. (Ed.). (2002). *Recognizing diversity in aging, moving toward cultural competence. Generations 26.*

Yeo, G. & Gallagher-Thompson, D. (Eds.). (1996). *Ethnicity & the dementias.* Washington, DC: Taylor & Francis.

Cross-Cultural Perspectives in Thanatology: Through a Prism of Religious Faiths

Monica Nandan, PhD

SUMMARY. Recent decades have witnessed an increase in thanatology education in colleges and universities. However, the infusion into thanatology curricula of religious faiths as they affect behaviors, experiences and emotions of dying individuals and survivors is still in its infancy. In this article I describe an effective approach I have used to integrate various religious beliefs and practices into an undergraduate course on death and dying. Before presenting my approach, I provide a brief description of the state of death education in professional and undergraduate institutions in America and a rationale for infusing cross-cultural components into thanatology curricula. *[Article copies available for a fee from The Haworth Document Delivery Service: 1-800- HAWORTH. E-mail address: <docdelivery@ haworthpress.com> Website: <http://www.HaworthPress.com> © 2005 by The Haworth Press, Inc. All rights reserved.]*

KEYWORDS. Thanantology, education, cross cultural comparison, diversity, cultural competence

Attitudes toward, and meanings attributed to, death and dying are culture bound. Aries (1981) and Illich (1990) have traced the cultural

Monica Nandan is Associate Professor of Social Work and Coordinator of Gerontology Program, Department of Government, Social Work & Sociology, Missouri Western State College, 4525 Downs Drive, St. Joseph, MO 64501 USA (E-mail: nandanmo@mwsc.edu).

[Haworth co-indexing entry note]: "Cross-Cultural Perspectives in Thanatology: Through a Prism of Religious Faiths." Nandan, Monica. Co-published simultaneously in *Gerontology & Geriatrics Education* (The Haworth Press, Inc.) Vol. 26, No. 1, 2005, pp. 43-56; and: *Aging Education in a Global Context* (ed: Dena Shenk, and Lisa Groger) The Haworth Press, Inc., 2005, pp. 43-56. Single or multiple copies of this article are available for a fee from The Haworth Document Delivery Service [1-800-HAWORTH, 9:00 a.m. - 5:00 p.m. (EST). E-mail address: docdelivery@haworthpress.com].

Available online at http://www.haworthpress.com/web/GGE
© 2005 by The Haworth Press, Inc. All rights reserved.
doi:10.1300/J021v26n01_04

meaning of death in Western thought from the Middle Ages, when death was considered natural, to the present, when it has become something "alien" that happens in intensive care units of hospitals. According to Dickinson, Sumner and Durand, "[m]ore dying occurs 'offstage' today in hospitals and nursing homes . . ." (1987, p. 58). Rinpoche (1995) and others projected that Americans would be entering yet another stage in the cultural meaning of death by adopting a holistic attitude toward this phenomenon. Rinpoche suggested that while practical and emotional care may be adequately provided for dying individuals and their survivors, their spiritual needs will have to be met by exploring the meaning of death and life.

Cultural sensitivity and cultural competence are essential to meet the needs of dying individuals and their families from a great variety of backgrounds (Irish, Lundquist, & Nelson, 1993). The Educational Work Group of the International Work Group on Death, Dying and Bereavement recommended that in preparing professionals in health care and human services, death educators must "promote awareness and sensitivity to distinctive needs and responsibilities of the diverse populations to be served" (International Work Group on Death, Dying and Bereavement, 1991, p. 238). Therefore, graduates of various professional health and social service programs (e.g., social work, psychology, medicine, and nursing) must become knowledgeable about and sensitive to how terminal illness, death, and grief affect individuals from diverse ethnic and religious groups with whom they will work (Parry & Ryan, 1995).

There is scant literature on the current state of death education in undergraduate and professional schools, and even less information on how to infuse cross-cultural contents into thanatology curricula. Through this paper, my intent is to bridge some of the gap by describing an innovative approach that I used to integrate a cross-cultural component into an undergraduate course on death and dying. I describe this approach against a backdrop of the state of death education in professional and undergraduate institutions in America, and I also provide the rationale for infusing cross-cultural components into thanatology curricula.

STATE OF DEATH STUDIES

Death is an inescapable aspect of each person's reality. Across time and culture, [people] have devised a variety of ways of handling the psychological, social, economic, and political consequences of death and the process of dying and of grieving (Kalish & Reynolds, 1976, p. 187).

Herman Feifel, the first modern death educator, spearheaded the death awareness movement in the 1960s. Elisabeth Kübler-Ross's publication in 1969, *On Death and Dying*, further fueled an interest in death studies (Doka, 1985). Since then, significant effort has been made to refine death education programs in America (Wass, 2004). Death education initiatives have developed from elementary to graduate schools (Dickinson et al., 1987; Morgan, 1987), with support for academic and research efforts by organizations such as the Association for Death Education and Counseling (ADEC) (Crase, 1989). A cursory examination of leading death-related journals–such as *Death Studies* and *Omega*– and various text books clearly indicates the large number of disciplines and professions that are interested in, and contribute to, this topic (Crase, 1989).

In a survey of 1,251 colleges and universities, Cummins (1978) found that 75 percent of these institutions were offering courses on death and dying through 62 different departments. Since the 1970s, discussion on death and dying in undergraduate liberal arts courses in such disciplines as religion, philosophy, psychology, gerontology, and art has steadily increased (Coppola & Strohmetz, 2002; Crase, 1989; Dickinson, Sumner, & Frederick, 1992; Hill & Stillion, 1995; Stefan & Coll, 1978), though until recently, less than desirable discussions have occurred in medical, dental, nursing, and social work schools (e.g., Alexander, 1990; Bertman, 1988; Duont & Francoeur, 1988). Professional schools or programs that offered a separate course on death and dying did so mostly as a one-credit course (Duont & Francoeur, 1988). A few studies about thanatology in professional schools (e.g., Dickinson et al., 1992; Downe-Wamboldt & Tamlyn, 1997; Duont & Francoeur, 1988) found that the topic of death and dying was mostly offered either as an elective or as a component of a core course for medical and social work students. For instance, for social workers, content on death and dying was weaved into a course titled "Human Behavior and the Social Environment" or into a gerontology course (Dickinson et al., 1992). A more recent study of medical school curricula dealing with end-of-life issues revealed an increase of such course content between 1975 and 2000. In 2000, palliative care was directly addressed in 87 percent of over 200 medical schools responding to a survey, and the majority of students in these institutions were exposed to information about hospice care (Dickinson, 2002). Especially since 1998, training programs for physicians, such as "Education for Physicians and End-of-Life Care," have created separate death education courses in nursing schools and an

End-of-Life Nursing Education Consortium was established in 2000 (Wass, 2004).

The extent and level of infusion of thanatology into professional and liberal arts curricula still leaves a lot to be desired (Dickinson et al., 1992). This desire is clearly evidenced in the avoidance and ambivalence in our society about death. For instance, in mainstream American culture, talking and learning about death customs is either avoided or, in any case, not common-place. Euphemisms are used to continue to keep the "D" (death and dying) words out of our daily parlance and lexicon. Instead, words such as "end-of-life," "palliative care," and "patients who are life threatened" are commonly used in the medical and social service community today (Wass, 2004, p. 303).

CROSS-CULTURAL INFUSION INTO THANATOLOGY CURRICULA

Thanatology courses in American undergraduate and professional schools normally address the following topics within a Western context: suicide, attitudes toward death, death anxiety, patterns of grief, mass death, terminal illness, death at different ages and due to various causes, hospice, dying in institutions, funeral rituals, and beliefs about life, death and life-after-death. Each of these dimensions of death and dying could be assumed to be viewed and experienced in a different fashion in the various cultures and subcultures that make up the United States of America. Consequently, a middle-class, heterosexual, Anglo-Saxon approach to grief delineated in the classical thanatology texts (e.g., Kübler-Ross, Saunders, Worden, & Parkes, c.f. DeSpelder & Stickland, 2005) may not be relevant in multi-cultural contexts such as the U.S.A. For instance, in cultures that strongly believe in life-after-death, the reactions of survivors could be very different from those who do not have similar beliefs (Parry & Ryan, 1995).

Hence, teachers of this subject in undergraduate and professional schools in the U.S. should incorporate cross-cultural contents to make their students sensitive to the culturally diverse clientele they can be expected to serve (Irish, Lundquist, & Nelson, 1993). Educators can instill the importance of cross-cultural education in thanatology by treating culture as a major thread that runs through all aspects of end-of-life experiences, rituals, communication, and decisions (Doorenbos, Briller, & Chapleski, 2003). The method, depth and breadth of integration of this content into graduate and undergraduate courses could certainly vary.

Ideally, in these courses any or all of the dimensions of death and dying discussed above could be examined from the perspectives of any number of major ethnic groups and faiths, given the fact that the United States comprises not only multi-ethnic but also multi-faith based groups. According to the 2000 U.S. Census, over 30 percent of its population was non-White, with recent immigrants predominantly originating from Mexico, India, China, Philippines, Vietnam, El Salvador, Cuba and Haiti. Additionally, Americans identified themselves with 35 different Christian denominations and 20 different religions (e.g., Jewish, Muslim, Buddhist, Unitarian, Hindu, Scientology, Baha'I, etc.) from across the world (U.S. Census Bureau, 2003).

American society is not a single, homogenous entity with just one death system and one universal set of death-related encounters and attitudes. On the contrary, our society embraces within its boundaries a kaleidoscope of cultural, social, racial, ethnic, and religious groupings, each of which may have important differences in some aspects of their death-related experiences (Corr, Nabe, & Corr, 2000, p. 103).

The meaning of death is similar in some respects and varies in others across cultures (Rosenblatt, 1993). Even in the United States, the meaning of death for a Creole, a Navaho, a Lutheran, a Catholic, a Muslim, a Jew or a Buddhist could vary systematically (Atchley, 2000). Moreover, there are many intra-ethnic and intra-religious group differences in perspectives on, and practices related to, death (Grollman, 1993). For example, death rituals vary across India, with different practices in south and north India. Similarly, the rituals surrounding a Catholic death in India most likely would be different from that in the U.S. because of the different contexts. Invariably, the host culture influences the faith that is imported, such as Catholicism–imported to the Indian sub-continent through missionaries–was influenced by the Indian culture.

Cultures deal differently with end-of-life decisions such as advance directives, resulting in varied completion rates of such a document. For instance, for Korean-Americans, family decision-making may be more highly valued than an individual's expression of treatment preferences because in this culture the smallest unit of care is the family and not the individual. The notion of autonomy is perceived through a sociocentric rather than an egocentric lens. Similarly, among African-Americans–with the notorious Tuskegee syphilis study still a haunting memory–there is widespread mistrust of the health care system. As a result, African Americans may perceive the signing of an advance directive as tantamount to signing away their rights (Beresford, 1999).

Generational differences in values and practices may also come into play. For example, second-generation immigrants may not share the values of their parents, and this may cause tensions especially related to end-of-life decisions. Mental health, health care professionals as well as social service workers can unwittingly add to the emotional distress and suffering of bereaved family members if they are not sensitive to the values and culture of the dying person (Lickiss, 2003). Practitioners should be sensitive to cultural elements such as female modesty in Islamic practices, unique religious practices such as *santeria* of Cubans, Korean cultural norms about touching and eye contact, the meaning of family among Native Americans, family roles and priorities of Puerto Ricans, cultural barriers to health care among Arab-Americans, and the importance of courtesy in Hmong culture (Parry & Ryan, 1995).

Being culturally competent includes, but is not limited to, communicating and disclosing the imminence of death sensitively to the dying person and his/her family, understanding the modes of decision making in a specific family context, understanding the disease and its symptoms within the cultural context, learning about the different ways of conceptualizing death and dying, customs surrounding death, burial/cremation, attitude toward medication, therapy and nutrition, privacy issues and spiritual matters (Lickiss, 2003). Becoming culturally competent in death-related matters about different ethnic and religious groups in the U.S., though, is exceedingly difficult for students in health and human service programs without appropriate training. However, if these students are introduced to a sampling of faiths with different beliefs and practices related to death and dying, they have a better chance of becoming practitioners who are at least sensitive to cultural diversity. Such training will also make them feel comfortable in seeking additional information on groups with whom they interact most frequently. As practitioners, they can then learn more about specific groups, or know whom to ask and what to ask, so as to alleviate some of the emotional pain of dying persons and the survivors by interacting in a culturally sensitive or culturally competent fashion with them. As one medical professional noted: We [in the medical professions are] willing to devote years to learning the technology and how to handle it. Why wouldn't we be willing to spend a few months learning about how to care for the soul of that person who happens to have this disease and is dying? (Kagawa-Singer, c.f. Beresford, 1999, p. 3).

INCLUSION OF CROSS-CULTURAL COMPONENT INTO DEATH AND DYING COURSE

In this section I describe the cross-cultural course contents of an undergraduate course titled "Death and Dying" taught within a gerontology program. This format for integrating culture could easily be employed in professional schools that teach courses on death and dying. I have been teaching this course for over ten years during which time the format has evolved, with more emphasis being placed on the cross-cultural components. Doubtless, there is more than one effective or appropriate way to teach this subject matter, but the approach I sketch here has some especially effective features that others teaching this material might want to adopt. To facilitate this adoption, I first describe the characteristics of students who typically enroll in the course. I then briefly outline the concept of culture as it relates to the objectives of the course. Finally, I describe the assignments for a cross-cultural project and a panel presentation, evaluation criteria, and learning outcomes.

Most students who enroll in this course are in their junior or senior year and come from a wide range of majors including, but not limited to, education, business, psychology, social work, nursing, physical therapy, and mortuary science.

To communicate the nature and importance of culture, I explain to my students that culture encompasses ethnicity, gender, age, religion, spiritual practices, and several other dimensions (Doorenbos, Briller, & Chapleski, 2003). For example, what one considers "common sense" is determined by culture and thus quite variable across cultures. Culture is a system of shared ideas, concepts, beliefs and rules that shape how people experience life and death (Queralt, 1996). Culture is like a photographic lens where different lenses can create different kinds of images. Culture is a strong determinant of a people's views of the very nature and meaning of illness and death, of how end-of-life decisions can or should be controlled, how news about death should be communicated, and how other related decisions should be made. In other words, attitudes toward dying, death, spirituality and religion are invariably integrated into the belief systems of all cultures.

The fear of death drives many people to turn to religion because of its potential to diminish fears through rituals, customs, healers, priests, and other spiritual specialists (Parry & Ryan, 1995). For many individuals, religion plays an integral part in coping with dying and grieving. Therefore, the first objective of this course is for undergraduates to learn how different religions impact dying and death, and to compare and contrast their beliefs and practices. The second objective is to afford students an opportunity to develop new perspectives after they have evaluated the diversity of death-related practices and beliefs through the following assignments.

One vehicle for achieving this objective is a cross-cultural project which consists of a paper and a panel presentation. I list in my syllabus at least a dozen religions or faiths such as Buddhism, Jainism, Confucianism, Catholicism, Scientology, Hinduism, New Age, and others for students to choose from, though they may, with my approval, research a religion not on the list. Additionally, I provide students a list of criteria they need to address as they research the death and dying beliefs and practices of the faith they chose. Specifically, they need to identify the following aspects of that faith: (i) beliefs about a Higher Power, personhood, death, life and the afterlife; (ii) rituals performed during the dying process, at the time of death, and after death; (iii) rituals demarcating the transition from life to death; (iv) attitudes toward Western medicine and the meaning of such principles as autonomy and self-determination; (v) traditional funeral rituals; (vi) method of disposing of the body and concomitant rituals; (vii) attitudes toward the death of young people compared to that of older adults; (viii) role of women during funerals and roles of other immediate family members after death; (ix) norms for mourning and grieving, and (x) practices marking death anniversaries. Students may add other relevant aspects.

As the class discusses these topics throughout the semester, students share their research findings, providing a variety of perspectives on the topics under consideration. By discussing a wide range of perspectives during the semester, students clarify concepts, share their reactions and thoughts, and identify beliefs and behaviors surrounding death and dying. They have time to reflect upon the significance of beliefs and attitudes of people from different faiths and in turn even modify some of their own beliefs and attitudes. These discussions nurture student growth in self understanding and respect for others very different from them.

At the completion of their research project, students participate on a panel. Students who have selected religions characterized by more similarities than differences are placed together on a panel. Students are required not only to present relevant key aspects of the religion they studied but also to create an environment that depicts and evokes the faith that they are presenting by bringing to class artifacts such as clothes and food, videos, music/chants, inviting guest speakers who are of the faith, and by drawing on web sites for descriptions and illustrations. Students start by providing a brief overview of the faith to contextualize their presentation about death-related customs and beliefs.

An important pedagogical strategy I use is to encourage students to compare and contrast death and dying experiences across faiths. In a post-panel discussion, students identify similarities and differences in attitudes, beliefs, practices and customs of the various faiths that were presented by panelists. They also gain an understanding of the wide-ranging attitudes toward Western medicine and the ethical principles that guide people from various faiths. For instance, students contrast attitudes pertaining to invasive surgery or blood transfusion held by Jehovah's Witnesses with those held by Protestants. Students make similar comparisons between Hinduism and Zoroastrianism regarding beliefs about life-after-death.

This exercise enables students to recognize death as a common experience for all humans, while developing sensitivity to the differences in experiences and practices across the globe. A significant revelation that students share during their panel presentation is their recognition of intra-faith variations in practices and customs even if beliefs may not vary significantly. For example, students have discovered that Catholic practices surrounding death vary in Mexico, the United States and India, because the respective ethnic cultures interact with the faith to create a distinct set of customs surrounding death and dying. To convey such instances of syncretism, students make their case by providing illustrative examples.

While the research that students conduct allows them to gain a thorough understanding of one religion, panel presentations expose the whole class to all the other faiths students have studied. Comparing and contrasting elements across faiths forces students to further analyze each faith and thus achieve a higher level of understanding of cross-cultural differences and similarities. In addition to revealing intra-faith differences in practices across the globe, panel presentations often reveal more similarities across faiths than students might have expected.

I evaluate the cross-cultural papers for students' comprehensiveness in addressing the research criteria listed earlier, clarity of writing and for number of references utilized in the document. Criteria for evaluating presentations include the following: quality of handouts, degree of preparedness for the presentation and mastery of the topic (reading the paper to the class is unacceptable), creativity in presentation and use of audiovisual materials and artifacts. Over the past ten years most students received a grade of B or higher for this assignment because they turned in several drafts of their papers during the semester and rewrote the final document based on my feedback and comments; rewriting strengthened the quality of both their papers and presentations.

In reviewing students' written end-of-semester feedback received over ten years, I identified the following quotes from seven students as fairly representative of general student reactions to this exercise:

> "I gained some new insight into the religion that I chose to [research] as well as insight into other faiths chosen by the panelists in class. The open discussions following the panels made the class very interesting. There is so much to learn from other faiths across the world about how to live our lives."

> "The panel made the class that sounded morbid into a well rounded class from which I learned a lot and I enjoyed it too."

> "The panel allowed us to discuss a 'taboo' topic so much more openly."

> "The atmosphere created by the panelists for their respective religions helped me understand the faith better and address some of my stereotypes."

> "When I first started conducting my research on the Muslim religion, I thought I already had a pretty good grasp [on] this religion [because of my brother-in-law]. While I already knew about some of the religious beliefs of the Muslim [community], I didn't understand why Muslims had these beliefs. This assignment gave me a deeper understanding to the question of why Muslims perform certain tasks (e.g., making the once in a lifetime pilgrimage to Mecca), and avoid certain foods (pork and liquors) and why these things are so important to the Muslim people and the Muslim culture. . . . After completing this research assignment I believe I could explain to anyone why Muslims perform certain tasks, why these tasks are important to Muslims and how they feel it will affect them spiritually if they do not perform these tasks. Before this assignment I would have never felt confident enough to speak about another religion. I would have been too intimidated. I also would have been afraid of misinforming someone, or unintentionally passing on stereotypes about this religion especially as it pertains to dying and death issues."

"[The panel-based overview of the various faiths and death related practices] will save me valuable time by [my] not having to learn about the different aspects of the many different religions I may encounter as a professional. While I still don't know everything about every religion, I now have a strong basic understanding of approximately 14 different religions that, before this assignment, I had little or no knowledge about. [Because of the panel presentations] I feel [that] I may not embarrass myself or my clients [during a very sensitive event in their lives]. I did my research paper . . . on Judaism [and this project prepared me to some extent] for my career in nursing. . . . [During] the first semester of nursing school we were taught that [it] is very important to consider cultural preferences of patients at all times. . . . [This semester] as a Patient-Care Tech at a local hospital, I had the opportunity to use this knowledge about people of Jewish faith. The nurse was shocked that I knew so much about [a particular family at the hospital] and remarked how much easier it made the process of dying for [our patient]. . . . When I graduate and become a hospice nurse, this knowledge about the Jewish faith will be very useful [as will the knowledge about all the faiths] and I am appreciative of all the different faiths shared during our panel. . . . I think all nursing students should have to take this course."

"I was exposed to a Multicultural Panel in which the ideas, beliefs, and customs of a variety of faiths were discussed relating to death. The panel ranged widely, representing diverse faiths and beliefs from Wicca to Hindu to Latter Day Saint. The experience impacted me greatly. By gaining knowledge about diverse beliefs relating to death, I was better able to create my own concepts of death, grief, and the afterlife. Furthermore, as a future social worker, I feel this knowledge will benefit my work with clients, as I will be less apt to look at clients in an ethnocentric manner. Instead, due to the awareness of differing beliefs and norms gained through the multicultural panel, I will better equip myself and my clients with the tools necessary to help them in times of grief and mourning."

CONCLUSION

Death as a topic for discussion, research, and socialization in the United States emerged during the 1970s but experienced a renaissance of interest during the 1990s. Schools and colleges are currently teaching or discussing death more than they did in the 1970s (Dickinson et al., 1992). Although death education in universities is expanding–relaxing the cultural taboos concerning discussions of death, and increasing professionalization of death education–much is still wanting in this field (Wass, 2004). Since the topics of dying and death are not the exclusive domain of any particular discipline, Ratner and Song (2002) recommend that all colleges and universities either offer a general course on dying or integrate material on death and dying into the curricula of as many disciplines as possible, or both. Additionally, colleges and universities could prepare health care professionals to better serve their multicultural clientele in situations of dying and death by putting more emphasis on teaching culturally appropriate behaviors towards terminally ill patients and their families.

I have incorporated cross-cultural elements into the death and dying course that I teach at my institution. Each student in this course researches one faith/religion and at the end of the semester he/she presents the findings pertaining to its beliefs, practices, customs, death artifacts, and other relevant aspects. Since the presentations are made in a panel format, students become culturally sensitive about at least a dozen different faiths through presentations made by their class mates, and culturally competent in at least one faith–the one they researched. During the panel presentations students pool their lists of references which become an excellent resource for work with dying individuals from diverse backgrounds. Generally, this teaching approach prepares students to be less likely to judge or stereotype people from different faiths as they experience death and dying.

REFERENCES

Alexander, R. (1990). Concepts of thanatology in the nursing curriculum. *Loss, Grief & Care*, 4(1-2), 7-11.

Aries, P. (1981). *The hour of our death*. New York: Knopf.

Atchley, R. C. (2000). *Social forces and aging: An introduction to social gerontology* (9th ed.). Belmont, CA: Wadsworth Thomson Learning.

Beresford, L. (1999). Cultural differences last a lifetime: Tailoring end of life care to a diverse population. *ABCD Exchange*, March, http://www.abcd-caring.org.

Bertman, S. L. (1988). The thanatology curriculum at University of Massachusetts Medical School. *Loss, Grief & Care*, 2(1-2), 57-64.

Coppola, K. M., & Strohmetz, D. B. (2002). How is death and dying addressed in introductory psychology textbooks? *Death Studies*, 26, 689-699.

Corr, C. A., Nabe, C. M., & Corr, D. M. (2000). *Death and dying, life and living* (3rd ed.). Belmont, CA: Wadsworth/Thomson Learning.

Crase, D. (1989). Death education: Its diversity and multidisciplinary focus. *Death Studies, 13*, 25-29.

Cummins, V. A. (1978, September). Death education in four-year colleges and universities in the U.S. Paper presented at the first *National Conference on the Forum for Death Education and Counseling*, Washington, DC.

DeSpelder, L. A., & Strickland, A. L. (2005). *The last dance*. Boston: McGraw Hill.

Dickinson, G. E., Sumner, E. D., & Durand, R. P. (1987). Death education in U.S. professional colleges: Medical, nursing, and pharmacy. *Death Studies, 11*, 57-61.

Dickinson, G. E., Sumner, E. D., & Frederick, L. M. (1992). Death education in selected health professions. *Death Studies, 16*(3), 281-289.

Dickinson, G. E. (2002). A quarter century of end-of-life issues in U.S. medical schools. *Death Studies, 26*(8), 635-646.

Doka, K. L. (1985). The crumbling taboo: The rise of death education. *New Directions for Student Services, 31*, September, 85-95.

Doorenbos, A. Z., Briller, S. H., & Chapleski, E. E. (2003). Weaving cultural context into an interdisciplinary end-of-life curriculum. *Educational Gerontology, 29*(5), 405-416.

Downe-Wamboldt, B., & Tamlyn, D. (1997). An international survey of death education trends in faculties of nursing and medicine. *Death Studies, 21*, 177-188.

Duont, E. M., & Francoeur, R. T. (1988). Current state of thanatology education in American health professions and an integrated model. *Loss, Grief & Care, 2*(1-2), 33-38.

Grollman, E. A. (1993). Death in Jewish thought. In K. J. Doka, & J. D. Morgan (Eds.), *Death and Spirituality*. New York: Baywood.

Hill, L. J., & Stillion, J. M. (1995). An interdisciplinary undergraduate seminar: "Death and dying in psychology and theater." *Death Studies, 19*, 365-378.

Illich, I. (1990). *Limits to medicine*. New York: Penguin Publishers.

International Work Group on Death, Dying and Bereavement (1991). A statement of assumptions and principles concerning education about death, dying, and bereavement for professionals in health care and human services. *Omega, 23*(3), 235-239.

Irish, D. P., Lundquist, K. F., & Nelson, V. J. (Eds.). (1993). *Ethnic variations in dying, death and grief*. Washington, DC: Taylor and Francis.

Kalish, R. A., & Reynolds, D. K. (1976). *Death and ethnicity: A psychocultural study*. Los Angeles: University of Southern California Press.

Lickiss, J. N. (2003). Approaching death in multicultural Australia. *Palliative Care, 179*(15), S14-S16.

Morgan, M. A. (1987). Learner-centered learning in an undergraduate interdisciplinary course about death. *Death Studies, 11*, 183-192.

Parry, J. K., & Ryan, A. S. (Eds.). (1995). *A cross cultural look at death, dying and religion*. Chicago: Nelson-Hall Publishers.

Queralt, M. (1996). The *social environment and human behavior: A diversity perspective*. Boston, MA: Allyn & Bacon.

Ratner, E. R., & Song, J. Y. (2002, June). Education for the end of life. *Chronicle of Higher Education. 48*(39), B12.

Rinpoche, S. (1995). *The Tibetan book of living and dying.* London: Rider.

Rosenblatt, P. C. (1993). Cross-cultural variation in the experience, expression and understanding of grief. In D. P. Irish, K. F. Fundquist, & V. J. Nelson (Eds.), *Ethnic variations in dying, death and grief.* Washington, DC: Taylor and Francis.

Stefan, E. S., & Coll, F. (1978). Perspectives on death: An experimental course on death education.

U.S. Census Bureau (2003). *Statistical Abstracts of the United States: 2003*(123rd ed.). Washington DC: Government Printing Office.

Wass, H. (2004). A perspective on the current state of death education. *Death Studies, 28*(4), 289-308.

Heroes of Their Own Stories: Expressions of Aging in International Cinema

Robert E. Yahnke, PhD

SUMMARY. This study of 14 international feature-length films (1988-2003) is aimed at providing gerontologists with models of successful aging that portray elders as being valued within the context of community. Elders serve as role models and mentors for the young, and they resolve mid-life crises for the middle-aged. Elders complete their life's work in the context of community (aging in place), where they struggle to maintain abiding values and draws others to the community. The study concludes with examples of key visual metaphors utilized at the endings of selected films that affirm the role of elders as catalysts for change for the young, the middle-aged, and even their communities. *[Article copies available for a fee from The Haworth Document Delivery Service: 1-800-HAWORTH. E-mail address: <docdelivery@haworthpress.com> Website: <http://www. HaworthPress.com> © 2005 by The Haworth Press, Inc. All rights reserved.]*

KEYWORDS. Aging in film, aging in place, community, intergenerational relationships, mentors, mid-life crises, role models, wisdom

---

Robert E. Yahnke is Professor of Film & the Arts, The University of Minnesota, 258 Appleby Hall, 128 Pleasant Street S.E., Minneapolis, MN 55455 (E-mail: yahnk001@umn.edu).

[Haworth co-indexing entry note]: "Heroes of Their Own Stories: Expressions of Aging in International Cinema." Yahnke, Robert E. Co-published simultaneously in *Gerontology & Geriatrics Education* (The Haworth Press, Inc.) Vol. 26, No. 1, 2005, pp. 57-76; and: *Aging Education in a Global Context* (ed: Dena Shenk, and Lisa Groger) The Haworth Press, Inc., 2005, pp. 57-76. Single or multiple copies of this article are available for a fee from The Haworth Document Delivery Service [1-800-HAWORTH, 9:00 a.m. - 5:00 p.m. (EST). E-mail address: docdelivery@haworthpress.com].

doi:10.1300/J021v26n01_05

Aging across the life course, in international cinema, is based upon three straightforward themes: childhood and adolescence is a time for mentoring by elders; middle age is a time for resolving mid-life crises (with the assistance of elders), and old age is a time for expressing one's wisdom and equanimity through contributions to the wider community. In other words, the life course in international cinema is based upon the strengths and positive values of active elders, who are an integral part of family and community contexts. The films analyzed below focus on elders who either have been agents of transformation or have been refined and transformed, often in the context of community. The films portray older adults who are almost always valued as *elders* within their communities.

At every stage of life–youth, middle age, or old age–individuals face challenges and transitions that propel them forward toward a greater sense of personal and psychological wholeness or well-being. In the first two stages of life–youth and middle age–the old often serve as mentors or guides, helping to resolve crises, assist in significant passages or transitions, and affirm and support the personal development of their charges. Such assistance is particularly significant in the context of mid-life crises. When international films portray elders apart from these two roles–as mentors and problem-solvers, what role is left for the old? In those cases, rather than facing new challenges that require them to overcome emotional and psychological crises in old age, elders in these films usually demonstrate the characteristics of courage, endurance, equanimity, and harmony as they respond to loss and finitude. Although they may not be perfect beings, their emotional lives are represented as being complete and their spiritual lives stripped down and simplified to their *essence*. In other words, the aging process that has taken them from childhood to adolescence to middle age to old age has granted them stability and serenity in the face of life's challenges. In all of these cases, the indomitable character of elderhood is illustrated most fully as oneness with community, especially as it is represented in the theme of *aging in place*.

Research in gerontology contains few studies of cinematic representations of old age in either American or international cinema. Some research has focused on images of aging in film (Flynn, 1989), gender (Hollenshead, 1977; Trojan, 1980), or theme (Cole, 1991). Other research has focused on portraits of aging in the context of educational film and videos (Yahnke, 1985, 1988, 1989). Over the years more than 30 reviews of feature-length films–including half that number that are international films–have appeared in the *Audiovisual Reviews* column of *The Gerontologist*. Some of these reviews have been organized thematically; for example, as Aging, Intergeneration & Community (Yahnke, 2000) and Old Age and Loss (Grabinski et al., 2003). One included brief reviews of several films (Yahnke, 2003). Another source for brief reviews of international films is an annotated bibliography, *Audiovisuals*, published by the Association for Gerontology in Higher Education (Grabinski & Yahnke, 2004). A comprehensive study of both educational videos and feature-length films combines analysis of American and international films that addresses themes of intergeneration and regeneration (Yahnke, 2000). These analyses emphasize the variety and complexity of the experience of aging. Likewise, this essay on international cinema conveys an essential set of universal themes about aging as they are expressed within a global context. These themes–of elders mentoring in intergenerational relationships, elders resolving mid-life crises, and elders expressing wisdom and serenity in old age–can be considered in the context of sociological, cross-cultural, demographic, and intergenerational research in global aging. Studying expressions of aging in international cinema may offer relevant and complementary perspectives on these avenues of research in global aging.

This essay highlights the contributions of 14 international films on aging that appeared between 1988 and 2003. These films offer students of global aging an opportunity to comprehend the experience of aging from the elder's perspective. Film has the power to convey complex, three-dimensional images of old age. In international films about aging, character determines plot. Character is inextricably entwined with the experiences, judgments, and values of the past; the characters' present circumstances and conflicts; and their insights into the limits of the future. The best plots are the ones driven by character change and personal transformations. The audience should care about the characters; and the film's plot should reveal the characters' strengths and weaknesses. Feature-length films offer much greater complexity of characterization, an in-depth illustration of significant themes relevant to aging, and subtle and complex interaction among characters. At the same time, the structure of the screenplay, the use of significant visual metaphors, the contribution of sound and musical themes, the technical strengths of the art of the shot or the art of editing, and the power of actors to realize three-dimensional characters provide insights into the multiple levels of art that are brought to bear on depictions of the aging process. Films reveal the changes that occur gradually in the emotional and psychological development of aging individuals. Using film as an adjunct to theories about global aging can help students more clearly grasp the individuality and idiosyncrasies of old age. Although it is difficult to integrate feature-length films into historical, cultural, and social-scientific educational contexts, gerontologists should have a basic understanding of the ways film communicates in the context of global aging. This article is meant to provide teachers and researchers with that understanding.

The first section of analysis below, *Elders as Mentors*, portrays elders as positive role models for the young and the middle-aged. In these films elders are willing to adapt, to take a stand, and even to sacrifice for the younger generation. These films promote the mutual benefits of intergenerational relationships: elders assist the young and the young support and affirm elders. The second section, *Elders Resolving Mid-Life Crises*, illustrates the significant roles that elders play in the lives of the middle-aged (especially when those individuals face mid-life crises). Elders interact with characters in middle age whose emotional, psychological, and spiritual selves are unresolved. These characters face one or more internal conflicts they need to resolve; and the process of the film is to put those characters into motion–guided by the sure hand of elders–to see whether or not their conflicts can be resolved. In the context of the narrative tradition of film, that motion takes on the metaphor of a journey in which individuals struggle to resolve their emotional and psychological pain. The third section, *Elders in Community*, affirms the capacity of elders to refine the meanings of their own lives and achieve a measure of wholeness, self-understanding, and harmony in their old age–especially in their having contributed to the continuity of traditions in a variety of community contexts. International films about aging make the sense of place (neighborhood, village, or city) a character–and in that sense portray the identities and values of the old as grounded in the context of their communities. The metaphor of *aging in place* signifies that the community acknowledges that elders are significant links to traditions and rituals and play an important role in maintaining the continuity of those values on behalf of the community. The fourth section, *Images of Intergeneration and Community*, expands upon ideas analyzed in the other sections by focusing on significant visual metaphors–either based upon intergenerational relationships or upon elders as change agents within communities. The way these films end express a simple truth: the old are the heroes of their own stories. Each of these concluding scenes sums up the ways in which elders are the catalysts that enable the young and the middle aged to complete key transitions in their lives; at the same time, the images of elders in community portray old age as a time for an attainment of wisdom, expressed through courage, hardihood, equanimity and serenity (Yahnke & Eastman, 1995).

ELDERS AS MENTORS

In many international films childhood and adolescence are a time for mentoring by the old. In these films the young receive life lessons from the old. Often the old are surrogate parents and play a significant role in the young person's emotional and social development. For instance, in *Cinema Paradiso* (Italy, 1990) Alfredo, an old man in a Sicilian town, mentors a child whose father died on the Russian Front in WWII. Alfredo is the projectionist in the town's cinema, and he befriends Toto, who is fascinated with movies and eventually becomes his assistant. Like a father, Alfredo listens, advises, protects, and affirms. In adolescence, Toto experiences his first love, and Alfredo responds with compassion and insight when he realizes that Toto has fallen in love with a woman from a different class. Alfredo subtly tries to persuade Toto that he should look elsewhere for love.

Likewise, an old woman tries to help a boy find his father after his mother is killed in an accident in *Central Station* (Brazil, 1998). Dora is a retired schoolteacher, scraping by financially by writing letters for illiterate travelers in Rio de Janeiro's Central Station. At first, her compassion for the boy Josuè is motivated by the desire to assist him in finding his father. But as the two embark on a long journey into the interior of the country, searching for the boy's father, her role becomes more complex. The two form a strong intergenerational bond. Dora helps the young boy resolve his grief over his mother's death, and when it appears that they will not be able to find Josuè's father, she offers to be his surrogate parent and form a permanent bond.

The mutual benefits of intergenerational relationships are also evident in *Central Station*. Although Dora and Josuè do not establish a family unit after all, Dora's interaction with him leads her to a powerful insight into her own unresolved past. By helping the boy find his father, Dora is reconnected to her own memories of her father, and after years of not facing her unresolved feelings about her father, in the climactic scene of this film she is able finally to address them in a letter she writes to Josuè.

The plot of *The King of Masks* (China, 1996) carries forward the idea of surrogate parenthood and also affirms the mutual benefits of intergenerational relationships–but with a significant plot twist. An old street performer in 1930s China, known as "the king of masks," seems content to perform with a monkey as his assistant. But how will he pass on his craft to another generation? Once he had a son, but the boy died when he was only 10 years old. A chance encounter with a famous opera star spurs the old man to find an heir, someone he can tutor. In a run-down neighborhood of town, he purchases an eight-year-old boy from one of his parents. Street urchins are everywhere because of the overwhelming poverty of the era, and parents are willing to sell one of their children so they can buy food for the others in their family. When the old man hears the boy address him as "Grandpa," he is moved, and later–when he learns the boy has been abused–the emotional bonds between the two deepen. But then comes the plot twist–the *boy* is revealed to be a *girl*. Initially the old man rejects her, and then reluctantly takes her on as an employee (treating her the same as he treated his monkey assistant). Eventually, the old man's heart softens when he realizes the extent of the girl's courage and devotion to him. Then the old man teaches her his art–in defiance of everything he has come to believe in this patriarchal culture.

Spring, Summer, Fall, Winter . . . and Spring (South Korea, 2003) also portrays an intergenerational relationship based upon the transmission of a set of values from one generation to another. The entire film takes place on a tiny Buddhist monastery built on a raft in a lake. One monk resides in the monastery, and at the beginning of the film he has one novice–a small boy who lives with him. Where did the boy come from? The answer is revealed only at the end of the film–after the boy has grown into an adolescent, run off with a young woman brought to the monastery by her mother for physical and emotional healing, returned to the monastery years later after murdering his wife in a jealous rage, leaving with police to be taken to prison, and then returning in middle age after being released from prison. In that last season another woman brings a child to the monastery and leaves him behind–so that he will have a better life than she can offer him. Now we realize that the first young boy in the early scenes was another orphan, left to be raised by the resident monk. So one intergenerational bond yields to another intergenerational bond, and the role of the elder again is to provide physical, emotional, psychological, and even spiritual support for the younger generation.

Franco Zeffirelli's *Tea with Mussolini* (Italy, UK, 1999) illustrates how multiple mentors can impact a young person's personal development. Inspired by the story of Zeffirelli's own upbringing, the film tells the story of a group of women expatriates from England, known as the

Scorpioni, who have formed a tight-knit community in Florence. One of them, Mary Wallace, accepts the task of raising a young boy, Luca, after he is abandoned by his father and deposited in an orphanage. Luca is one of many children who are born out of liaisons between married men and their lovers. Mary Wallace is the most practical and down-to-earth member of the group, and she arranges a complicated schedule with her friends to provide Luca with a liberal education. One of the most memorable scenes in the film is Mary Wallace teaching Luca Shakespeare's *Romeo and Juliet* by having him construct a puppet theater and reading the balcony scene using paper puppets. The creativity of the teaching exercise, the intimacy between teacher and student, and the magic of Shakespeare's language makes the scene come alive. Her lesson: "True love lasts forever. It's the most important thing." In effect, Luca's experience affirms that it takes all of the *Scorpioni* (the *village* in the context of this film) in order to raise a child.

In *Antonia's Line* (Holland, 1995) the title character returns to her old village at the end of WWII with her adolescent daughter and sets about establishing her own extended and diverse family, including neighbors that were abused by their family members, a defrocked priest, an abandoned woman and her children, and a widower and his sons. In effect, this strong-willed matriarch raises her own village. "No one seeks her help and protection in vain," a character says about her in one scene. Antonia creates her extended family–her *line*–and she defends it at all costs so that it may be perpetuated through time. Antonia is a woman of the earth, a farmer, someone who connects her days and nights to the rhythms of the seasons, the turning of the sun and the moon, and the processes associated with living and dying. She makes no moral judgments about life and death. In a conversation with her great-granddaughter Sarah near the end of the film, she asserts, "Nothing dies forever. Something always remains from which something new grows. So life begins, without knowing where it came from or why it exists," and she concludes by saying, "Life wants to live."

Since Otar Left . . . (France, Belgium, 2003) is another example of how elders fearlessly sacrifice for the young so that they can thrive in ways that were not open to the older generation or to the middle generation. In this film, an old woman, her daughter, and her granddaughter live a meager existence in a decaying neighborhood in Tblisi, Georgia (a former Soviet republic). The old woman's hope for the future is pinned upon Otar, her son, who is living in Paris and studying medicine. Eventually, word comes that Otar has died, but the two younger women conspire to keep Otar's death a secret from the old woman, Eka–because they fear she will she will not be able to bear the tragedy. Eventually, Eka surprises both when she announces that she has sold her invaluable library of French literature, assembled by her late husband, arranged for visas for all three women, and bought tickets to Paris so they can visit Otar. In Paris the old woman confirms what she had expected–that her son is dead–and yet she keeps that discovery to herself. When all three are at the airport, and ready to board their plane back to Georgia, the old woman drops hints to her granddaughter to stay behind in the lounge. With her visa in hand, the young woman will be able to stay in Paris. Since Otar is dead, Eka wants Otar's legacy passed on to the next generation–to her granddaughter. The old woman takes charge in the face of a family crisis and surmounts all obstacles in order to determine the truth of Otar's disappearance and then to sacrifice for her granddaughter, so that she can have a better life.

Mentoring can even occur when an elder is not physically present–in some respects–for that mentoring. For instance, in *Yi Yi: A One and a Two* (Taiwan, Japan, 2000), an adolescent is stricken with guilt when her grandmother suffers a massive stroke at home. The granddaughter is afraid her grandmother was completing an errand she was responsible for, and she cannot forgive herself for that lapse in judgment. After being hospitalized, the grandmother is sent home in a coma, and the physician encourages the family to take turns sitting in the grandmother's room and reciting their daily activities. Although family members try, soon they give up–thwarted by the one-sided character of the interaction. Near the end of the film, the young woman returns home, after suffering a serious emotional crisis, and finds the grandmother sitting up in a chair next to her bed. She kneels next to her grandmother and puts her head in her grandmother's lap. Their interaction is serene and peaceful. She thanks her grandmother for forgiving her at last, and she asks–with a new perspective born of the suffering she has experienced, "Grandma, why is the world so different from what we thought it was?" She adds, "Now that you're awake, and see it again, has it changed at all?" Then the girl falls asleep in the old woman's lap. The cut to the next shot shows the granddaughter asleep in her own bed. She has been dreaming, and through her dream she found the consolation she required. Even though the old woman was in a coma, she was still the elder of the family, and her granddaughter still needed her affirmation and approval in order to overcome her emotional crisis.

In each of these examples, elders play significant roles in helping the young make the transition from either childhood to adolescence or from adolescence to adulthood. The old listen, inspire, teach, affirm, accept, sacrifice, and challenge the young to let go of the past, resolve old hurts, form new and diverse family bonds, accept their own shortcomings, and embrace new and unsettling ways to view the world.

ELDERS RESOLVING MID-LIFE CRISES

In international films about aging, middle age is filled with self-doubt and a lack of self-confidence. Characters are stuck in middle age, and they need help in order to resolve their emotional and psychological crises. If they were mentored by elders when they were young, now they need them again to be affirmed, consoled, or guided through the perils of mid-life crises. In international films on aging the central metaphor of middle age is the mid-life crisis, and the primary means of resolving those mid-life crises falls to the elders in their lives.

For example, *Cinema Paradiso* (Italy, 1990) depicts three aspects of the life course of the main character Salvatore. We see him as a child, an adolescent, and as a middle-aged man. But the entire film is told from the point of view of the middle-aged Salvatore, after he learns (in the film's second scene) that an old mentor of his, Alfredo, has died. Suddenly Salvatore slips into crisis mode. We learn that he has not returned home since he was a man in his early 20s. Since then he has become a successful producer of films and is highly regarded for his cinematic achievements. Alfredo was a surrogate father figure in Toto's childhood and a wise uncle or grandfather-figure in Toto's adolescence. But all that Alfredo has done for Salvatore is incomplete until the middle-aged version of our main character returns to this childhood home to attend Alfredo's funeral.

When Salvatore returns home and revisits old haunts, he realizes that everything Alfredo did for him was meant to set him free. The last time he saw Alfredo alive was when he left his small town and took the train to Rome. Alfredo's advice to him: "Don't come back. Don't think about us. Don't write. Don't give in to nostalgia." So many things have not changed in the small village. Salvatore's mother has even maintained a shrine to his childhood in his bedroom. But one other thing has not changed: Salvatore has never gotten over losing his first great love in adolescence. But what can Alfredo do now to help him through his mid-life crisis? After all, Alfredo is dead. The answer comes with a final gift from Alfredo–given to Salvatore by Alfredo's widow. Alfredo's final gift is a compilation of movie clips he assembled over the years; and every clip shows passionate scenes of lovers kissing in a variety of films–all from Salvatore's youth in the cinema. A flood of memories assaults Salvatore as he watches the clips. Even now Alfredo is speaking to him through this gift–and his message to his beloved Toto is to let go of the past, let go of that long-lost love, and live again with the passion expressed in all of these scenes. As Salvatore watches the clips unfold, he begins to relax and cry–and he begins a process of self-forgiveness and emotional healing. His reaction to this gift suggests that even in middle age it is not too late to receive a life lesson. Alfredo is brought to life again by his final gift to Salvatore; and in this final visitation he is able to convey once more his affection for his surrogate son as well as guide him through a particularly difficult mid-life crisis.

An elder son's return home in *Shower* (China, 2000) precipitates his mid-life crisis, which is resolved to a great extent by his father's wisdom and insight into human nature. In many ways the elder son is a stranger to his father. He lives in a large metropolitan area, and he is a successful businessman. His father, in contrast, runs a traditional bathhouse in an area of a city that is targeted for urban renewal. Initially, the elder son endures a chilly reception from his father, and that alienation is made worse when that son fails to take care of his developmentally disabled younger brother while running an errand. The father lashes out at the elder son about his lapse in filial piety.

But the friction between the two is resolved one night when the elder son wakes up in the middle of the night during a rainstorm and discovers that his father is up on the roof trying to nail plastic sheeting over the windows. The elder son joins him, and after a wordless greeting, the father and son get down to business and nail the sheathing. Later that morning, they sit on the roof and look out over the other houses in the aging neighborhood. The son notices that the houses are the same as the ones he knew as a child. "Houses are like old people," his father says. "No matter how hard you try to fix them up, they're still old." But then he adds, "They're still special." For the first time in the film the father and son share a moment of intimacy. The elder son has gained an insight into his own past, and the bonds of filial piety are strengthened by this interaction. Eventually, after the father's death, the elder son commits himself to caring for his younger brother. Now he is able to fulfill the obligations of filial piety, and he embarks upon that task without complaint because he has been transformed by his return to his expected role within the family.

In *Minor Mishaps* (Denmark, 2002) a family's life is thrown into crisis when the mother dies unexpectedly. The three adult children (two daughters and a son) assume that the father is vulnerable now and requires careful tending. The truth is that the mother was the glue that held the family together; now that she is dead, each is a planet in its own orbit. All three of the adult children carry on; but they are barely surviving– as each faces his or her mid-life crisis. But all roads lead back to the father, the one calm and emotionally stable person in this family. After he survives a health crisis, and the family is gathered around him, the old man tells them, "We can talk about minor mishaps, but not death." The father is going to make it. The family is going to make it. And as the film ends, each of the family members resolves his or her mid-life crisis because of his secure and affirming guiding touch.

In *Spring, Summer, Fall, Winter . . . Spring* (South Korea, 2003) a middle-aged man returns to a tiny Buddhist temple in the middle of a remote lake in the mountains. An old monk is the sole occupant of the temple. The middle-aged man once lived there as a child and as a young man, before he ran away with a young woman. In fact, this old monk was his surrogate father. Why has he come back now? We learn that he has escaped from the police after being arrested for the murder of his wife. In the section entitled *Fall* the old monk calms the escaped man and slowly begins to focus the man's energies so that he will be able to take personal responsibility for his actions. The old man paints hundreds of large Chinese characters on the wooden platform of the temple, and–as a form of penance–he asks the younger man to use his murder knife to etch those characters into the wooden floor. The man works for days to finish this task, and when the police catch up with him, the old monk makes them wait while the murderer completes his task. Then they take him away. The monk's commands are all about spiritual laws; he is interested in his former student finding repentance and forgiveness before he is removed from the monastery and punished in the secular realm. In the world of this film an individual can be restored to wholeness only if the physical actions are in harmony with restorative, psychological, and spiritual justice. The old monk's wisdom sets the stage for the murderer to return to the monastery after serving his sentence and then carry on the work of his former mentor.

Yi Yi: A One and a Two (Taiwan, Japan, 2000) begins with a wedding and ends with a funeral. Both scenes emphasize the uncertainty of a moment of passage–in the first case, the uncertainty of a new marriage bond, and in the second case the closing of one intergenerational set of relationships in a Taiwanese family that has survived an emotional and psychological crisis. When a grandmother suddenly suffers a massive stroke, and is left in a coma, her family begins to disintegrate. The old woman's daughter is unable to sit at her mother's bedside and talk to her each night; she flees to the sanctuary of a religious community. A granddaughter is stricken with guilt because she blames herself for the old woman's illness; her life is thrown into turmoil upon a failed first love. The old woman's son-in-law, N.J., is able to sit comfortably with the unresponsive old woman and tell her what is on his mind. Eventually he shares the terms of his mid-life crisis when he admits, "There's very little I'm sure about these days."

One of the most interesting relationships in the film is between N.J. and a Japanese businessman called upon to "rescue" their company. This man is middle-aged, but older than his years in many ways. He is more *sensei* than businessman; in fact, he believes one can be successful in business only if one acts in accord with spiritual laws. The businessman is drawn to N.J. immediately because he realizes N.J. is an honest and humble man. After a dinner together, the Japanese businessman concludes simply, "You are a good man." The Japanese businessman acts the role of the *elder* by recognizing N.J.'s talent, singling him out for his positive values, and trusting him to make good business decisions. At the end of the film, after revisiting his first great love, N.J. returns home just before the grandmother dies. N.J. and his wife, who has returned from her sojourn in the religious community, sit and talk about their recent crises. N.J. admits that he was reunited with his former lover. But he tells his wife that he learned a significant life lesson: "Even if I was given a second chance, I wouldn't need it." Finally he is able to let go of the past. He realizes he must leave his business partners because they no longer share a common set of values. He knows that he must honor the bonds of his marriage and family. He has returned home restored and rejuvenated, and two *elders* in his life–his mother-in-law and the Japanese businessman–have guided him to this place of healing.

Thus, elders are needed as guides and mentors even for those in middle age. Their accrued wisdom and experience is brought to bear upon mid-life crises just as they are upon the trials of youth. These films reveal the willingness of the old to help the middle generation resolve unfinished business, let go of nostalgia for the past, accept new and challenging roles, reconcile intergenerational disputes, redeem themselves from self-imposed exiles, and restore long-suppressed emotional entanglements. In all respects these interactions between the middle aged and the old are transforming and rejuvenating for characters trapped in middle age.

ELDERS IN COMMUNITY

In most international films aging in place has a set of positive connotations. The old play a vital role in their communities. They are valued as "elders." They are repositories of stories, memories, rituals, and traditions. They know the old ways. They love the land, and they are committed to maintaining their connections to the land. Along the way they have struggled to maintain a sense of "community," drawn the young to them, functioned as mentors, and passed on their values to future generations. They have survived poor crops, deaths, disasters, and wars. Aging in place is a central metaphor for a personal fulfillment in old age.

In *Shower* (China, 2000) an elder son, a prodigal son, is the one who left the old ways behind, moved to a new city, and prospered. He is the modern Chinese man–cell phone always at the ready. When he visits his father, Master Liu, he returns to a tight-knit community that is the hallmark of aging in place. His father runs a traditional bathhouse, frequented mainly by elders, and he is well and happy walking the well-worn ruts of this humble life. He sums up the contentment of old age when he tells his son, "I can eat, I can sleep, and I can work." The old man's wisdom is integrally connected to the metaphor of aging in place. He is at one with the routines of the bathhouse. He cares for his younger, developmentally disabled son, and he has fostered a set of harmonious relationships with his regular customers. Inevitably he faces the loss of this community because of the increasing pressures of urban renewal. At the core of the film is a serious message about the ways in which community provides continuity and harmony in one's life, and the way in which filial piety–even in the context of a caregiving crisis–can transform a person and contribute to a sense of personal redemption.

If the bathhouse is the core of the community in *Shower*–receiving men of all ages and social ranks for hours of social intercourse–then the pub is the center of the community in *Waking Ned Devine* (Ireland, 1998). The community gathers in the pub for meals and drinks, and members of the community spend hours gossiping and telling stories and measuring the world against community standards. In this context old people are a regular part of daily social intercourse. This film suggests that old age is the time of life to be savored for its sweetness, a time to assume new roles, a means of maintaining continuity for the community. The experiences of four old friends in *Last Orders* (United Kingdom, 2001) highlight another example of the pub as the metaphoric center of the community. Four men have spent their youth, middle age, and then their old age as pub regulars. The pub is the center of their social life and their neighborhood. Each major developmental step in their lives has been announced and/or lived-out in the context of the pub. When one of the four dies, the remaining three friends face changes and new challenges in their old age–and all three meet first in the pub to organize a final farewell to their friend.

Babette's Feast (Denmark, 1988), based on a story by Isak Dinesen, and depicts an outsider's integration into community. The film portrays a small commune of elders, members of a dwindling religious sect, who have aged in place in a remote village on the coast of Norway. They welcome into their midst a refugee from Paris named Babette. She labors for years as their cook, and she ages in place with the others. She becomes a valued member of the community because of her excellent cooking skills, her financial acuity, and her self-effacing behavior. The climax of the film occurs when Babette serves the elders of this community a special meal. The meal is practically a religious experience, a subtle and yet heartfelt form of communion and it has the power to transform the others around the table. Members of the religious sect–who throughout the film have devoted themselves only to things of the spirit, and not of the flesh–turn to each other and admit to past wrongs and deceits. The others accept those admissions without making any judgments. Later, in the sitting room, sipping coffee and champagne, several members bless the others and call across the room, "Dear Brother" or "Dear Sister." Two members even turn to each other, kiss affectionately, and then stare endearingly into each other's eyes. What magic has been brought upon this community of elders! Outside in the open air they are all smiling, they all take each other's hands, and they dance and sing around the well in the yard. As they separate, one of the men leans against the well, looks up into the starry night, and concludes, "Hallelujah!" Babette's feast is a triumph of the heart over the head. For one night, and with one meal, a community of elders is affirmed and restored by her compassion, selflessness, and artistic skill.

The community formed in *Antonia's Line* (Holland, 1995) also is expressed through the metaphor of meal as a form of communion. In this film a widow returns to her family farm after WWII with her teenaged daughter. Early in the film, after Antonia has begun to draw some of her neighbors to her, they celebrate with a wonderful feast at a long table in Antonia's front yard with Antonia seated at the head of the table. This scene is the first example of what becomes a metaphor for all that Antonia is able to accomplish in the film–establish a matriarchal community. In that sense, the family dinners in the front yard of Antonia's farm represent the extended family that will become Antonia's line. The meal is a communion of sorts, based upon Antonia's spirit of kindness and tolerance. If *Babette's Feast* was the story of one woman's power to transform a small community of diners, then *Antonia's Line* documents one woman's power to restore an entire community and its embedded patriarchal values. If Babette is the consummate artist, then Antonia is the paradigm of the matriarch.

Since patriarchy is based upon bloodlines, the line in Antonia's case is based upon her willingness to take in a diverse set of individuals into her family unit. In short, Antonia *assembles* her line person by person throughout the years of her life. In one respect she assembles a family that extends to three generations before she dies; but this family broadens to become a tight-knit community, and this community becomes a reflection of all that is good in the matriarch Antonia: her kindness and tolerance, her affection for all members, her respect for others, her openness to new ideas and diversity, and her willingness to defend the community against external threats.

Eat, Drink, Man, Woman (Taiwan, 1994) is a final example of how meals function as metaphors for community. In this case the head of the community is an old widower raising three daughters. Every Sunday the busy family gathers around the table for a meal prepared by the father, a retired chef. His mealtime preparations are legendary, and the table always is filled with diverse dishes. But more important is that the Sunday dinners are times for sharing news and for marking transitions in everyone's life. Most of the film is about the daughters resolving their love lives. But an underlying theme in the film is that their father, in his old age, has reached a state of wisdom, patience, and self-understanding that holds the family together. The old man is always there; and his meals are a means of providing security and harmony in their otherwise hectic lives.

International films portray older adults who have functioned as mentors, aged in place, drawn people to them, and fought to maintain the values of their *community*. They have lived within the context of old traditions and unchanging ways. The old have been tested by experience; they are survivors, negotiators, and realists. The old have reached an understanding that the individual is nothing unless he or she is part of the community. In many international films old people participate in community, foster community–and even in some respects create community. Elders in these films complete their life's work in the context of community, and thus they either transform others or are themselves transformed through that process.

IMAGES OF INTERGENERATION AND COMMUNITY

Film is a visual medium, and some of the most significant images of aging in international films occur at the ends of the films when the intergenerational relationships are summed up through key visual metaphors that signify the bonds that have been created and/or strengthened through the action of the film. In every case elders are portrayed as having achieved a sense of harmony and serenity in light of those relationships. For instance, *The King of Masks* (China, 1996) ends with a still image of the old man and his adopted granddaughter–both smiling and content now that the terms of their relationships are resolved. The last shot in *Central Station* (Brazil, 1998) is a close-up of Dora, the main character, sitting on a bus, after she has left her surrogate son behind so that he can live with his new family (his two brothers). She writes a letter to the boy now, and she tells him how much she misses her own father–even now in old age. That last close-up of the old woman illustrates the extent of the suffering and loss in her life and yet underscores how much she has gained by helping the boy find his family.

Spring, Summer, Fall, Winter . . . and Spring (South Korea, 2003) ends where it began–with a scene of a middle-aged monk raising an orphan on a tiny monastery in the middle of a lake–just as he was cared for by a former monk when he was an orphan. Just as the film begins in *spring*, it must end in *spring*. This repetition reaffirms the metaphoric and spiritual implications of the cycle of life and the cycle of the seasons: both move from regeneration to fullness of life, to decay and death, and then on to regeneration.

The last shot in *Eat, Drink, Man, Woman* (Taiwan, 1994) shows a father and daughter sitting at the table in their home for the last time. Throughout the film, this table has been the site of Sunday dinners, where the family gathered to share news and experience communion as a family unit. Now the old widower's three daughters have sorted out their lives, and he is ready to move on and sell the old family home. In this scene his daughter (who inherited his skills as a chef) cooks for him for the first time, and he is overjoyed because for the first time in the film he can taste the food. She stands next to him at the table. He holds up his bowl. Suddenly he says, "Daughter," and she responds, "Father." Through the communion of the meal the two have reconciled themselves and expressed an essential image of an intergenerational bond.

Several films utilize the ending scene to illustrate the powerful bonds of community, and the elder's place within that framework. For instance, in the last scene of *Waking Ned Divine* (Ireland, 1999) many of the members of the small community gather at the cliffs along the sea to toast the memory of their benefactor Ned Devine, an old man who died with a winning National Lottery ticket in his hand. Now the entire town will share his wealth. The townspeople bring the pub out of doors, and everyone toasts the old man–as if symbolizing the traditional Irish Catholic wake that is meant to commemorate the beginning of the soul's passage to heaven. What began for two old men in the village as an ill-conceived plot to gain riches has now helped them learn from their folly and gain wisdom; in effect, now they can taste the sweetness of life in this community, even though that sweetness has been tinged by loss.

Tea with Mussolini (United Kingdom, Italy, 1999) ends with a scene that reinforces the bonds between young man and the old women that raised him. As Allied forces mass just outside the hilltop village where the *Scorpioni*–the closely-knit group of elders–reside, the Nazis decide to blow up some of the towers in the city before they retreat. But one of the old women comes to the rescue and defies the commander. She entwines herself around the wiring to the explosives and prepares to die for her ideals. Just as the commander holds up his pistol to shoot her, another of the old women arrives on the scene and defies him too. "Stop this nonsense at once!" she fumes. She tells him she is shocked that he would even consider "blowing up old ladies!" All the other *Scorpioni* entwine the blast wires around their bodies. Of course, they carry the day, and when the Allies arrive, the young man they raised is with them. He has served in the Resistance. Their defiant last stand–based upon their passion for history and art–sums up all that they taught their young charge, Luca, when he was a child. Now the leader of the group, Mary Wallace, can congratulate Luca for becoming "the perfect English gentleman!"

At the end of *Yi Yi: A One and a Two* (Taiwan, 2000) a death unites the family. In the last scene the parents and their two children are alone in a small building where a table holds the photograph of the grandmother. The father and his adolescent daughter sit next to each other. The mother sits nearby with their eight-year-old boy. Suddenly the father clasps his daughter's hand; both characters have gone through similar crises in the film–one that experienced (and lost) her first love, and one that revisited his first great love and realized that he did not want to pursue that relationship further. The son, a boy of eight, approaches the table and reads aloud something he wrote when he finally thought about the meaning of her death. He tells his grandmother, "You always said you felt old." But then he mentions his baby cousin, still in the hospital. "I want to tell him I am old, too," the grandson says. Each of the four members of this family faced a crisis after the grandmother's stroke. Now. they are unified within the scene, and each has attained insights they lacked at the beginning of their trauma. Viewers can sense that this family unit has been strengthened by what they were able to survive. Each has an insight into the way people are broken by grief; and yet at the same time each has an insight into the powerful bonds of filial piety.

In the last scene of *Last Orders* (United Kingdom, 2001) a man's adult son and three of his friends arrive at the quay in Margate, England, to fulfill his wish that his ashes be scattered upon the water there. The highlight of the last scene is an image of three of the men huddled around the fourth, who removes the cover of the plastic urn and holds it out so that the men may reach inside. Each man digs into the ashes and then casts handfuls out into the sea. They say, "Good-bye, Jack," "Bye, Dad," "Bye, Jack"–as each throws the ashes up into the air so that the wind can carry them away. Then they share a moment of silence. When the urn is empty, the men walk away and decide to stop at a pub for a pint. Having fulfilled Jack's *last orders*, and having resolved some of their own longstanding disputes with each other, now the men are able to resume their social interaction in a familiar locale–the neighborhood pub. With an important ritual completed, they resume the thread of friendship that has sustained them for so long.

Similarly, Antonia's daughter, granddaughter, great-granddaughter, and members of her extended family gather around her as she dies in *Antonia's Line* (Holland, 1995). Antonia looks out the window and sees the setting sun. The narrator's voice explains the old woman's thoughts. Antonia looks at her daughter and realizes she will express her grief through her art; she looks at her granddaughter and realizes she will view her death with scientific curiosity; but when she looks at her great-granddaughter, the narrator says, "And I, Sarah, her great-granddaughter, would not leave the deathbed of my beloved great-grandmother because I wanted to be with her when the miracle of death parted Antonia's soul from her formidable body." The last shot of the film is a close shot of Antonia, her head on the pillow, as she turns her head aside, closes her eyes, and dies. Sarah, the film's narrator, has told the story of her great-grandmother's line, the matriarchal line of a proud, intelligent, and hard-working woman. In this film the sweep of aging, from generation to generation, is told as a means of showing how the generations move on, each yielding to the next generation, each refining something from prior generations.

These international films on aging offer gerontologists varied, complex, and yet ultimately hopeful views of the aging process. A primary task for elders is to serve as mentors and guides, to assist in key transitions in the lives of others, and to affirm and uplift others in the process. Finally, old age is viewed as a time of stability and serenity. The old have arrived at a place of wholeness and resolution, and their character and identity are complemented by their valued place in the community. The emotional core of their stories is the love and wisdom that flows readily from old to young, old to middle aged, friend to friend, family member to family member, and generation to generation–always in the context of community.

LIST OF INTERNATIONAL FILMS ANALYZED IN THIS ESSAY

Antonia's Line (Holland, 1995)
Babette's Feast (Denmark, 1989)
Central Station (Brazil, 1998)
Cinema Paradiso (Italy, 1990)
Eat, Drink, Man, Woman (Taiwan, 1994)
The King of Masks (China, 1996)
Last Orders (United Kingdom, 2001)
Minor Mishaps (Denmark, 2002)
Shower (China, 2000)
Since Otar Left . . . (France, Belgium, 2003)
Spring, Summer, Fall, Winter . . . and Spring (South Korea, 2003)
Tea with Mussolini (UK, Italy, 1999)
Waking Ned Devine (Ireland, 1998)
Yi Yi: A One and a Two (Taiwan, Japan, 2000)

REFERENCES

Cole, T. (1991). Aging, home, and Hollywood in the 1980s. *The Gerontologist, 31*, 430.

Flynn, B. L. (1989). Images of aging: Twenty years of films about the elderly. *Sightlines*: (Spring) 4-8.

Grabinski, C. J., Vanden Bosch, J., & Yahnke, R. E. (2003). Old age and loss in feature-length films. *The Gerontologist, 43*, 136-141.

Grabinski, C. J. & Yahnke, R. E. (2004). Audiovisuals. In *AGHE brief bibliography: A selective annotated bibliography for gerontology instruction* [CD-Rom]. Washington, DC: Association for Gerontology in Higher Education.

Hollenshead, C. (1977). *Past sixty: The older woman in print and film*. Ann Arbor: Institute of Gerontology, University of Michigan-Wayne State University.

Trojan, J. (1980). Film portraits of aging men. *Media and Methods, 20,* 42-44.
Yahnke, R. E. (1985). Classic educational films on aging. *Minnesota Journal of Gerontology, 1,* 31-35.
Yahnke, R. E. (1988). *The great circle of life: A resource guide to films on aging.* Baltimore, MD: Wilkins & Wilkins.
Yahnke, R. E. (1989). Films that recreate the experience of aging: A new direction for gerontological education. *Educational Gerontology, 15,* 53-63.
Yahnke, R. E. (2000). Intergeneration and regeneration: Old age in films and videos. In T. Cole, R. Kastenbaum, & R. Ray (Eds.), *Handbook of the humanities and aging* (2nd ed., pp. 293-323). New York: Springer.
Yahnke, R. E. (2003). Reel images of aging: Reviews of recent films. *The Gerontologist, 43:* 603-607.
Yahnke, R. E., & Eastman, R. M. (1995). *Literature and aging: A guide to research.* Westport, CT: Greenwood Publishing Group.

Teaching Cross-Cultural Aging:
Using Literary Portrayals of Elders
from Chile and the United States

Barbara Waxman, PhD

SUMMARY. Literary texts are cultural artifacts revealing a society's values and attitudes; reading literature about elders and old age can change readers' ageist attitudes. Beginning with these assumptions, I discuss ways of teaching cross-cultural aging in undergraduate literature courses, using Chilean texts paired with American texts. Students learn how old age is socially constructed and how writers can either reinforce or challenge negative societal stereotypes of elders. Chilean texts reveal Chileans' respect and affection by associating elders with nature and ascribing to them otherworldly wisdom. American texts respectfully depict elders connected to nature, but not as transcending the earthly. *[Article copies available for a fee from The Haworth Document Delivery Service: 1-800-HAWORTH. E-mail address: <docdelivery@haworthpress.com> Website: <http://www.HaworthPress.com> © 2005 by The Haworth Press, Inc. All rights reserved.]*

Barbara Waxman is Professor, Department of English, University of North Carolina Wilmington, Morton Hall 132, 601 South College Road, Wilmington, NC 28403 (E-mail: waxmanb@uncw.edu).

The author thanks Dr. Paul Hosier, Provost of UNC-Wilmington, for funding her research trip to Chile in July, 2004, and Dr. Rene Venegas, doctoral candidate in linguistics at Catholic University of Valparaiso, Chile for sponsoring her research activities during her month in Chile.

[Haworth co-indexing entry note]: "Teaching Cross-Cultural Aging: Using Literary Portrayals of Elders from Chile and the United States." Waxman, Barbara. Co-published simultaneously in *Gerontology & Geriatrics Education* (The Haworth Press, Inc.) Vol. 26, No. 1, 2005, pp. 77-95; and: *Aging Education in a Global Context* (ed: Dena Shenk, and Lisa Groger) The Haworth Press, Inc., 2005, pp. 77-95. Single or multiple copies of this article are available for a fee from The Haworth Document Delivery Service [1-800-HAWORTH, 9:00 a.m. - 5:00 p.m. (EST). E-mail address: docdelivery@haworthpress.com].

doi:10.1300/J021v26n01_06

KEYWORDS. Cultural aging, literary elders, Chilean elderly, literary pedagogy, literary gerontology, social construction of aging

I am an English professor who had the good fortune to live and study in Chile on a Fulbright Grant in the summer of 2003 and to return there for additional research during July of 2004. During the first stay, I lived with a Chilean family in Vina del Mar. My Chilean family taught me about their culture's attitudes toward family, including the esteemed place of elders, by the respectful ways they interacted with their aged relatives and by the reverence with which they spoke to me of elderly relatives who had died. When I had only been in Chile two days, my host took me to meet his mother and his aunt. He seemed proud of them and also wanted me to pay my respects to them.

I wondered whether this deference toward elders is prevalent throughout Chilean society. If so, then what discourses cultivate Chileans' positive attitudes toward their old? My background in literature prompts me to speculate about how published literature, an important cultural artifact, reflects and shapes Chilean readers' beliefs about aging.

Like most English professors and literary theorists, I believe that literary texts give us access to a society's attitudes and values; that they also shape these attitudes and values. Theorist Louise M. Rosenblatt (1983) asserts literature's cultural function: "Literature acts as one of the agencies in our culture that transmit images of behavior, emotional attitudes . . . , and social and personal standards" (p. 223). Fredric Jameson, a Marxist theorist, adds that "narrative is not just a literary form or mode but an essential 'epistemological category'; reality presents itself to the human mind only in the form of stories" (Selden, 1989, p. 47). Through stories of later life, readers can grasp some of the real-life feelings and thoughts of the elderly and think about societal attitudes toward the elderly.

Kenneth Burke (1989) similarly posits that a literary text "singles out a pattern of experience that is . . . representative of our social structure" (p. 515). Careful readers will detect societal attitudes about old age conveyed through older literary characters and their stories. Literature becomes a tool to reveal the social condition of elders. Because, in Burke's view, reading is a form of doing, literature about aging also offers a way to "perform" or "try out" old age before we get there.

By bringing cross-cultural literary portraits of the old to the attention of students it helps to rectify the cultural invisibility of elders, and to remedy Americans' cultural illiteracy about later life (Woodward,

1991). Cross-cultural literary comparisons also uncover negative assumptions that students may have about elders. Examining the literature of aging cross-culturally enables students who have not traveled abroad to see how ageist attitudes are socially constructed and how writers either reinforce or challenge negative stereotypes of elders.

Finally, using this cross-cultural literature about elders in the classroom may change some students' ageist attitudes. Instead of offering our culture's master narrative of old age as loss, reduced productivity, and decline, some texts give readers what Hilde Lindemann Nelson (2000) calls "a counterstory" (p. 85). Margaret Morganroth Gullette (1997), in her study of the "midlife progress novel," discusses how these novels resist the narrative of decline and how their counterstories help readers to re-imagine their own middle and old age as a time of growth (p. 79). Students see the destructiveness of ageism because the literature persuades them to identify with elderly characters. Rosenblatt (1983) describes how students become more sympathetic through interactions with literary texts: "As the student vicariously shares through literature the emotions and aspirations of other human beings, he can gain heightened sensitivity to the needs and problems of others remote from him in temperament, in space, or in social environment" (p. 274). This quote applies to student-readers who learn through literature that young and old have much in common.

Zalman Schachter-Shalomi (1995), in his book *From Age-ing to Sage-ing*, written with Ronald S. Miller, pays tribute to the potential power of the arts when he envisions a new genre of "elder art," which will influence younger readers through its presentation of "images of older people that stress inner beauty, purpose, and radiance"; these images will help to create an attitude change: "Rather than having a horror of growing older, we will begin anticipating elderhood as the summit of life" (pp. 76-77). If the literature humanizes elders, then readers become humanely attuned to the lives of elders. Kathleen Woodward (1991) would agree. Reading literature about aging, she says, "can help shape the unacknowledged possibilities of our future experience in that largely unexplored realm of our cultural imagination–old age" (pp. 13-14).

Woodward's (1991) views reflect reader-response theory, which also guides my classes' analyses of literature. A certain kind of transaction between readers and literary texts–the "literary experience"–can transform readers, claims Rosenblatt (1983), the mother of reader-response theory. Reading is an active process in which readers create textual meanings, based on cues in the text in combination with their own unique knowledge, emotions, interests, and experiences. Rosenblatt

(1983) persuasively argues that "literature contributes to the enlargement of experience" during these transactions between reader and text: "We [average adult readers] participate in imaginary situations, we look on at characters living through crises, and we explore ourselves and the world about us, through the medium of literature" (p. 37). Implicit in this passage is the recognition that readers will identify with characters and situations that are skillfully drawn in literary texts. This identification broadens readers' understanding of others' experiences, offering insights into other people, other cultures, and other age groups.

The more intense the literary experience, according to Rosenblatt (1983), the greater the possibility of cultivating in readers humane values. She says that if students can have intense experiences of reading and discussing texts about elders, their ways of interacting with the elders may be permanently altered: "When there is active participation in literature . . . [one benefit is] the development of the imagination . . . the capacity to envisage alternatives in ways of life and in moral and social choices" (pp. 290-291). Student-readers of literature about aging might envisage a society beyond ageism.

With this view of the literary experience as my premise, I will discuss the use of cross-cultural literature about aging in the classroom to battle ageism. I have selected literature appropriate for a general humanities course such as Women in Literature or Approaches to the Study of Literature. This literature is also appropriate for gerontology classes where students may not have an extensive background in literature.

In this essay I argue that Chileans' traditional respectful and affectionate attitudes toward elders which I observed on a small scale is still evident in some of their modern literature. This respect has sometimes taken the form of ascribing to elders–especially old women–an almost mystical power that may grow out of their intimate relationship with nature. I consider here how to teach Chilean literature in juxtaposition with some American literature about later life. Usually I begin with poetry, grouping together a Chilean and an American poem about elders and nature. When we compare the Chilean poem with the American poem, students observe social constructions of aging and stereotypes of elders that the poems either reflect or resist.

I start my exploration with Chile's most famous literary son, the Nobel-Prize-winning poet Pablo Neruda. But before I do, I want to briefly provide a little more background on the place of elders, particularly female elders, in Chilean society.

ELDERLY WOMEN IN CHILE

I do not wish to romanticize the place of elders in Chilean society based on my observations of one family. Nevertheless, idealization of elders seems a part of the cultural discourse. For example, an article about Chile articulates the following view of elders' place in Chilean society: "Chilean families are very close knit and often include grandparents, aunts, uncles, and cousins. The elderly are respected and are cared for by their children" (*www.settlement.org/cp/english/chile/ family.html*). While in rural areas these traditional values and practices still are likely to prevail, in Chilean cities there are increasingly individuals who see elders living in their families as unproductive economic burdens, a view which a young economics professor suggested to me; adult children may also resent the respect and power they feel compelled to give the elderly parents who share their homes. If the elderly parents are affluent and the middle-class adult children are having financial difficulties, the adult children may also resent their continuing economic dependency on the parents. Finally, with more women in the workplace, families cannot give the elderly full-time care in their homes (De Vos, 1998). If they are affluent, they turn to *casas de reposo* (rest homes) for this care of their old relatives. These issues regarding the elderly, widely faced in the U.S., are surfacing in Chile as well. In a 1998 study of elderly unmarried women in Chile and Mexico, the author, Susan De Vos, found that both countries "could be considered on a threshold between having a more traditional and a more modern way of coping with a dependent elderly population" (p. 7).

I researched these notions about elders in Chile during my return visit to Chile in the summer of 2004. I interviewed my host family from the previous year, the host family of my colleague, as well as the family's maid, three students at Chilean universities, the three managers of the bed and breakfast where I stayed, five professors at Universidad Catolica de Valparaiso, and a tour guide in Iquique. This small sample does include people from both the middle and working classes.

One student from Universidad Catolica suggested there is a generation gap in Chile. She said emphatically that the old do not understand the young, their clothing, behavior, and lingo, and the young do not respect the old. Yet the teenage daughter of my host family would disagree, claiming that the young would not use bad language or disrespectful slang when among elders. I also noted quite a few times young men and women giving up their seats to elders (at 57 I was included in this category) on buses.

Moreover, my colleague's host "mother"–a middle-class or upper-middle class woman in her fifties, a homemaker, and her maid, a woman probably in her forties and of lesser education and lower class–both articulated the traditional view that elders are respected and taken care of in Chile. When Chileans turn to rest home care for relatives, they show some embarrassment and guilt for doing so and for seldom visiting (they are busy working to make ends meet). Four middle-aged adults stated these views about the homes: my host mother, one of our tour guides in Iquique, and two professors at Universidad Catolica,

One professor noted that the government is somewhat aware of the needs of older adults, making available to government workers upon retirement comfortable apartment complexes at Chilean beaches. In addition, there are community centers with programs for elders, classes at universities, and cheaper travel prices available to seniors. It seems Chileans are beginning to realize that the elderly population is rapidly increasing (9% were elders in 1998 and the percentage may grow to 23% by 2050, according to De Vos, 1998, p. 9) and that more provision needs to be made for them. Current provisions for elders seem to be mainly stopgap measures. Chile is, as De Vos, (1998) suggests, in transition from tradition to modernity. Perhaps the literary imagination can point to innovative ways of positioning elders in society and of caring for frail elders.

EXAMINING THE LITERATURE

A discussion of literary depictions of aging begins in my classes with short, accessible poetic texts. I pair Neruda's haunting poem, "Old Women by the Sea" ("Las Viejas del Oceano"; translated by Ben Belitt, (1966) with adjustments by me (pp. 300-303) and Theodore Roethke's "Old Florist." Roethke's brief poem describes an elderly male florist patiently tending and nurturing plants, watering roses all night, pinching back old petals, removing dead leaves; his power is especially evident in his ability to "fan life into wilted sweet-peas with his hat" (l. 9; Fowler & McCutcheon, 1991, p. 179). Neruda's poem describes an archetypal pilgrimage made by elderly matriarchs to the sea. The life-giving sea is the source of many supernatural Chilean legends, such as that of the *Caleuche*, a spectral ship steered by a demonic crew who are "eternally young" (Dorson, 1967). Class discussions uncover differences between Roethke's earth-rooted pragmatic old man and Neruda's oceanic, more ethereal old women (Belitt, 1966).

In Neruda's poem, the sea is described as violent and serious, forceful in its slashing motions and noisy trumpeting. The women, although "their fragile feet [are] broken" by the long journey of their lives, maintain their equanimity as they confront the sea. They have a strength that is unmoved by "terrorist waves." They are steadfast, awe-inspiring, sibylline, and courageous.

Because students tend to find poetry more challenging than other genres, I do a close reading of the poem with them stanza by stanza. As we do this, I ask students to consider the relationship between the poem's speaker and the women. The speaker reflects upon the women's origins, imagining that they are from our very own life-source and connected to human beings' past lives; they have touched and witnessed the eternal principle "in the fullness of time." So they have the power to claim the infinite ocean as their own, to "write signs" or "signatures" upon it that convey what life has taught them. The speaker's respect for these women increases with each succeeding stanza.

In the poem's final stanza, "the ancients" depart. Their contact with the infinite sea has "upraised" them, so they seem to ascend "on frail bird's feet." Their feet may be frail, but their presence has commanded a worshipful gaze. Their experiences and their connection to the sea have connected them to the core of human existence, enabling them to transcend time and enter the eternal realm. The speaker's tone is reverential as he reports their coming and going. After they depart, the traces of their influence remain. This poem is a strong example of the powers attributed to female elders in Chilean society.

Neruda's old women by the sea embody archetypal females, in particular the wise crone and the earth mother. By comparison, students learn that Roethke's florist does not convey a mystical or shamanic power; he is the wise, pragmatic elder, connecting with nature but not transcending it. One question for further discussion with the class is: how are old men and women represented in American fairy tales, folklore, and pop culture?

Chilean writer Adolfo Couve (2003) revises some of these archetypal associations of older women with the sea in his 1993 short story, "Seaside Resort." The version I discuss here is a translation by Katherine Silver. Rather than turning the old woman into an almost supernatural figure, Couve (2003) humanizes the protagonist, an elderly widow named Angelica Bow, through realism; setting her story in the seaside resort of Cartagena, he allows us to see her aging face and body, and even more important, to glimpse her fantasies and internal monologues. This story is comparable to British author Doris Lessing's (1984) *If the*

Old Could . . . , from *The Diaries of Jane Somers,* or to works by such American authors as Alice Adams and Alison Lurie (1998).

Before discussing Couve's (2003) story in class, I ask my students to answer some questions about the story's five-part structure, the narrator's methods of depicting the elderly female protagonist, the uses of the setting, and significant events in the story. I also ask them to express their reactions to the protagonist and to consider why they react as they do. Moreover, I ask them what they have learned about later life and female elders from this story. They answer these questions before we discuss the story in class.

Recent pre-discussion responses from students in two of my classes, "Approaches to the Study of Literature," suggest that the portrayal of Angelica usually evokes their sympathy and their pity, sometimes their respect for her lifetime of experiences; only one student out of more than forty reflects negative cultural and literary stereotypes of the old when she says that Angelica is bitter, angry, and nasty, like Miss Havisham in Dickens's *Great Expectations.* She and others express some unease at making contact with the elderly; the students fear their evident closeness to death as somehow contagious. Most of the students note Angelica's invisibility in the Cartagena social scene, her outmoded attire, and her rigid, empty routine. Her loneliness, sense of loss, yearning for companionship, and decrepit physical appearance not only elicit their pity, but also disturb and depress them. Two female students express fear of the physical aging process and of losing control over their environment; they confess that they prefer not to think about these unpleasant eventualities. Although these young women resist exposure to the foreign country of old age, they are a bit more prepared for it and for interacting with elders by having read this story.

Other discoveries about elders through the story are more startling for them. One student acknowledges having learned through the story that an elder may possess an entire life's history of good times and sad events, and that the old still experience the gamut of human emotions. What really amazes the majority, however, is that a female elder can still possess such avidity for life and that she may step out of her routine to take chances and make life happen. They are shocked at Angelica's sexual fantasies about young men–and at the notion that into old age the libido is still functioning. Ultimately, being privy to Angelica's desires, these readers understand how human she is; they identify closely with her. One young woman likens Angelica to her grandmother and speculates that Angelica could be herself a few decades in the future.

Clearly, then, many students do take an important lesson or two from this literary elder. Some admire the protagonist's avidness for life, her intense aliveness. And some who bring the assumption that elders possess wisdom and emotional stability to their reading of the story are surprised at the emotional turbulence displayed by Angelica. This character challenges the stereotype that emotional unrest is reserved for the young.

Nevertheless, fear is still the operative word that many of the students associate with old age–physical and emotional aging–in these responses. This fear needs to be confronted in class discussions of the story.

Primed by their responses to the pre-discussion questions, students enter into a lively discussion of the story. Class discussion often corroborates and strengthens many of the independent responses of students. The story can be discussed in class very systematically because of its well-delineated structure of nine pages divided into five sections. The class can be divided into small groups, each of which is responsible for discussing one section and for charting their reactions to the aged protagonist.

Readers view Angelica through the relentless gaze of the narrator; he writes with increasing intimacy of her aged body and demeanor. The skin on her thin bare arms hangs loosely, her hair is carefully coiffed and dyed, her dress has seen many seasons, her shoes and purse are passé, and her makeup is a heavy camouflage for her age. These aspects of Angelica are negatively described. What makes the narrator's gaze sympathetic, however, is how he also reports in the first section *her* gaze and *her* attitude: her eyes "impudently" watch the well-built men lounging on the beach. Her optimism is evident as she tells herself, "'if I am alive, it is impossible that nothing will happen to me'" (Couve, 2003, p. 86). Her inner monologue discloses that she is a life-affirming fighter who refuses "to capitulate" to the stasis of old age, to "her condition as an old woman" (p. 86).

The sea responds to Angelica's life-craving inner monologue with the affirming fluctuations of its waves. As Jack Tresidder (2003) reminds us, "The sea itself is the original source of life in many ancient traditions–a maternal image even more primary than the earth" (p. 50). Angelica connects with the sea, like Neruda's old women, and this contact nurtures her, rejuvenates her.

Something else that rejuvenates the protagonist is her sexual fantasies. These fantasies belie a stereotype of female elders as asexual. This stereotype may be more prevalent in the U.S. than in South America, and the difference merits class discussion about cultural constructions of old age. It does not usually occur to my students that Angelica may be a sensuous romantic who misses her husband sexually, so they need to be reminded about some symbolic objects in Angelica's bedroom. Her bedroom is perfumed by the two roses that she cuts from her garden daily: the roses and their fragrance suggest her romantic inclinations. Roses, especially red ones (no color is specified by the narrator), are associated with love, passion, and even women's genitalia (Tressida, 2003, pp. 228-229). Additionally, she still listens to love songs on the radio–crooned by a man with a seductive voice. She is ready for love.

Angelica is even prompted to remove her clothes and inspect her body in the mirror. This self-inventory, I point out to students, is a recurrent scene in literature about elders; Margaret Laurence's (1993) *The Stone Angel* and Doris Lessing's (1984) *The Diaries of Jane Somers* are two novelistic examples of self-appraisal in the mirror that records the "ravages" of time. What does Angelica find in the mirror, confirmation that her body is old, even though her mind may be youthful. The narrator describes "her flaccid breasts, her wrinkled belly, her ancient disproportionate shapes . . . thin legs and dyed hair" (Couve, 2003, p. 89). While she recognizes that her "body [is] devastated as if by a careless sculptor," the sculptor Time, yet she stands before the mirror and caresses her body, taking pleasure in her erotic fantasies; she is worthy of self-love and perhaps of love from others too. Woodward describes the literary portrayal of companionship with one's aged body in other texts: "[passages such as these suggest that] we may care for our body in old age as if it were a baby, *our* baby, paying attention to all its parts . . . [Often a] woman treats her body as a mother would her baby" (Woodward, 1991, pp. 176-177).

In American pop culture, sexualized elders are often the target of somewhat derisive humor, but in Couve's (2003) story, Angelica's fantasies are depicted with seriousness. I ask my class to consider the satirical ways in which the pursuit of love by old men ("dirty old men" primed with Viagra) and old women (seekers of young male studs) is depicted in our films and television shows. Are we more prudish or squeamish than Chileans about imagining sex among the geriatrics? The students do seem somewhat uncomfortable with the topic of geriatric sex. Yet geriatric sex is surfacing in popular shows on TV shows and in many feature films in movie theaters. These increasing depictions of sex between elders may make future student-readers of Couve's (2003) story less scandalized by Angelica.

Couve's (2003) story shows how Angelica's sexual fantasizing, first about a young plumber who comes to fix her bathroom and later about a man on the beach, makes her present and future seem sweeter. She takes pleasure in these erotic thoughts (p. 92); they feed her belief in the possibility of a change, of a miracle in her life. In class we discuss what is "normal" sexual behavior and fantasizing among elders and we note that, regardless of age, the most active sexual organ of the body is the brain. Angelica may be old, but she craves *eros*, not *thanatos*. And she is not the only literary elder to do so.

Sexual feelings are central to Doris Lessing's (1984) fictional story of Jane Somers's life as well. In *If the Old Could . . .*, Jane, a middle-aged widow, tells the story of her relationship with a middle-aged married man named Richard and describes the intensifying physical attraction between the two. Students are surprised that they are not the stereotypically reserved, or even prudish, Brits–and they are as hot-blooded as youths. Although the couples do not become lovers in the literal sense, Jane describes the powerfully charged, erotic atmosphere each time they meet. She notices the rejuvenating effects of these sexual feelings in her own body and mind; she feels the euphoria of a teenage girl in the throes of a "crush." Other stories of sexual affairs in later life can be brought into class, such as Adams's *To See You Again* and Lurie's (1998) *The Last Resort*.

By comparing Couve's (2003) story to Lessing's (1984), students learn that sexual fantasies and sexual vitality are not just for the young, that elderly women are not all asexual widows, affectionate grandmothers, and sterile old maids. Sexual behavior, they learn, is culturally constructed, but may also be culturally deconstructed through literature.

Finally, I turn to two nonfiction Chilean memoirs that include characterizations of elderly women, beginning with the work of a Chilean-Jewish writer Marjorie Agosin (2000). Her memoir, *The Alphabet in My Hands: A Writing Life*, contains affectionate portraits of her grandmothers and great-grandmothers. Although I have not yet taught Agosin's (2000) text in its entirety, these portrayals of her family's matriarchs have the power to change young readers' minds about the old, with whom they may assume they have nothing in common. The text works well with L'Engle's (1974) *The Summer of the Great-Grandmother*.

Before beginning discussion of the memoirs' portrayals of their elderly relatives, students should "freewrite"–write freely, nonstop, nonjudgmentally, without self-censorship–for a few moments about their own grandmothers. Often my Southern students have close relationships with grandmothers who live nearby, and they want to share with classmates their vivid sensory memories of visits with grandparents. They also have memories of deceased grandparents. We explore the significance of these memories in their lives. It is also useful to bring in portraits of older women done by artist Elizabeth Layton for discussion as well as magazine advertisements depicting elders, as bases for comparing Agosin's (2000) portrayals to those of L'Engle (1974).

L'Engle's (1974) account of her elegant Southern mother's descent into senility, with flashbacks to the prime of her mother's colorful life, is affectionate, but without the mystical presences of Agosin's (2000) portrayals. The narrative makes us privy to the author's problems as her mother's primary caregiver; we are given descriptions of her mother's nightmares, generalized fears, incontinence, and at times her rages at the author for being a "bad daughter" (Waxman, 1997). We witness how she copes with the erosion of her mother's personality by writing about her memories of the bright and vivacious mother she once knew. The narrative traces the author's work of mourning before and after her mother's death; she is comforted by her fervent Christian faith and belief in an afterlife. L'Engle (1974), finally, observes that her mother is fortunate to be surrounded by several generations of loving family members: hence her dying is a meaningful process.

Some students find this narrative of senility and death very unsettling. I ask students to consider not only the memoirist's strategies for enduring this alteration of her mother, but also to describe how they have dealt with it in grandparents or to imagine how they might deal with it in the future. I ask them to consider how L'Engle's (1974) depiction of her mother's senility may reinforce or dispel students' own fears about it.

In contrast to L'Engle's (1974) realistic portrayal of her mother, Agosin's (2000) discussions of her grandmothers and great-grandmothers are more reassuring for students. Yet what is reassuring about both narratives is that they represent the elderly matriarch in her youth as well as in old age. This enables readers to see the elderly person in context, as having lived a full life and as being an interesting person with a history. As Agosin (2000) describes her grandmothers and great-grandmothers, she remembers how they have shared memories of their own youth spent in Europe: Helena in 1930s Vienna during the rise of Nazism, and Raquel in Odessa. Agosin's (2000) narrative devotes much space to great-grandmother Helena, who had silently carried visions of "the sinister time" in Vienna (p. 59) and passes these along to Marjorie. The matriarch's European-Jewish origins invoke a mysticism which mingles with a Spanish-Indigenous-Chilean supernatural bent.

Folklorist Richard M. Dorson (1967), in his foreword to *Folktales of Chile*, notes that Chilean folklore reflects the beliefs, fears, and cultures of indigenous citizens, in turn influencing all Chileans. The folklore is peopled by evil spirits, sorcerers, animal characters, and witches. Yolando Pino-Saavedra (1967) observes that these tales are still being retold in Chile during wakes, at community work projects, and for children's entertainment (Pino-Saavedra, 1967). These tales often contain older characters that are culture-tenders or repositories of supernatural beliefs. Agosin (2000) mixes this multicultural Chilean folkloric material with Jewish beliefs and superstitions rooted in European folklore as she depicts the matriarchs of her family. This rich context provides students with a good basis for comparison to L'Engle's (1974) fervent Christian context. Students learn how literary depictions of aging and elders exist within a cultural and spiritual framework.

The dominant image Agosin (2000) uses to portray the matriarch Helena is a pair of Viennese candlesticks that hold the candles which she lights every Friday at sundown, to mark the beginning of the Jewish Sabbath. During the kindling of the lights, she prays for all humankind expelled from God's paradise (p. 60). As she lights the candles, Helena teaches her great-granddaughter that it is important to believe in angels and to imagine ourselves transported to "the ends of Sacred Eternity" (p. 60). Helena looks otherworldly, with a silver veil covering her "misty hair" (p. 60); and when lighting the candles, "she herself glowed with joy" (p. 60). Helena is shedding light on Marjorie, instructing her– as Agosin (2000) instructs readers through her description of Helena– about the role great-grandmothers often play in Chilean (or Chilean-Jewish) culture. Her role is that of culture-tender and spiritual leader of the family. Helena shows her granddaughter how to pray, and Agosin (2000) is grateful; she tells readers that "my prayers calm my spirit" (p. 60).

Students can readily see how this portrait of Helena is in contrast to that of L'Engle's (1974) mother during her irrational tirades and moments of fearful disorientation. I encourage the class to shut their eyes for a moment or two and summon up similar spiritual portraits of a grandmother like Helena singing in a church choir on Easter morning or lighting candles on Christmas Eve. I ask students to observe how these memories are culturally embedded in their own communities and families, and also how the memories operate against negative stereotypes of elders in the U.S.

The memoirist's visual memory of Helena exists beside an auditory memory of Agosin's (2000) great-grandmother Sonia, the deep voice of Sonia singing in Yiddish and "invoking guardian angels, invisible souls without names" (p. 63). Like Helena's mysticism during the lighting of

the Sabbath candles, Sonia's voice summons angels. Her singing peti-
tions the angels, messengers or ministers of God, for "life to grant us a
bit of luck" (p. 63). Sonia's singing in Yiddish, the European Jew's
mama loshen, or mother tongue, makes the spiritual content of the peti-
tion to the angels seem especially intense. In traditional Jewish liturgy
during Yom Kippur, the Holy Day of Atonement, angels become "independent beings whose task it is to transport the prayer of man to God, so
that He may have mercy upon the petitioner" (Encyclopaedia Judaica,
1972, p. 972). Most likely Agosin (2000) is appropriating angels from
Jewish tradition as literary figures to intensify the spiritual aspect of her
female relatives in her narrative.

Grandmother Hanna, also known as Chepi and Josephina, is the
daughter of Sonia and the matriarch whom Agosin (2000) confesses to
loving best. Chepi is Chilean-born, very wise, and flouts many of her
European mother's Jewish practices and views. But like the other old
female relatives, she is metaphorically associated with angels and pos-
sesses prophetic powers. The memoirist tells readers: "I know that she
is my guardian angel because she predicts dangers that lie in my path,
advises me to take care of my body, and her face appears to me during
hellish nights and in sweet dreams" (p. 65). Chepi hovers protectively
over Agosin (2000) and inhabits even her unconscious, her dream life.
The memoirist's bond with Chepi is evident when she expresses the fear
of losing her to death, because Chepi is so intertwined with her: Chepi
"is my memory, and if she ceases to exist, I might not know whom to
kiss or how to distinguish gestures of love and peace" (p. 65). Chepi is
the narrator's emotional barometer, her guide to the world of human
feelings, her link to her earliest affections.

Chepi is also Marjorie's guide to old age. When Agosin (2000) visits
Chile (Agosin now lives in the U.S.) to see 90-year-old Chepi, she observes in her not only time's effects, but also the centrality of memory to
elders' lives. She also witnesses Chepi's strong will to live (p. 181,
183). The memoirist reflects: "Perhaps that was the meaning of aging,
to let go of false belongings and to dedicate you to collecting moments
as if it were a breeze passing above the clouds or a garden of leaves in
the spirited crackle of winter" (p. 180). Claiming vivid moments and
living intensely in the center of these moments are central tenets of literature by and about the old–because their remaining moments on earth
are more finite. These collected moments are stored in Chepi's active
memory while her aged body stays "on night's final watch" (p. 182). I
ask students to freewrite about what they consider intense ways of using
time, of living in the center of the moment, and then to think about the

ways in which they waste their time. Literature about elders can teach the young to value time and to make contact with the core of most passing moments. Agosin's (2000) portrait of the wise Chepi shows students fearful of old age that many elders have developed the knack of living more fully in later life.

With Chepi's transition from memory and consciousness to forgetfulness, unconsciousness, and, finally, death, the author once again summons the imagery of angels to accompany her "to [her] final resting-place" (Agosin, 2000, p. 184). Her anticipation that "a young, frightened angel would at any moment carry her [frail Chepi] off" comes to pass (pp. 184-185). So vivid has been this portrayal of Chepi that student-readers are likely to mourn her passing and yet to feel her presence lingering mystically in their lives.

Another Chilean writer, Isabel Allende (2003), also reflects on aging in her recent memoir, *My Invented Country: A Nostalgic Journey Through Chile*. As the popular author–whose works have been translated into English by Margaret Sayers Peden and are widely read in the U.S., Allende's (2003) residence now–discusses Chile, she treats readers to affectionate, quasi-mystical portraits of her grandparents. Allende's (2003) elders, especially the women, are her muses; she confesses to writing "in a trance, as if someone was dictating to me, and I have always attributed that favor to the ghost of my grandmother, who was whispering into my ear" (p. 180). Like Agosin (2000), she clearly connects family with Chile itself: "blood ties . . . bind me, too, to my land" (pp. 22-23). Allende's (2003) memoir compares well to Agosin's (2000) for its mysticism; and Allende's (2003) mysticism combined with humor contrast to *The Summer of the Great-Grandmother*, with its serious examination of the psychological and practical problems faced by a caregiver of the elderly.

I begin discussion of Allende's (2003) text by asking students to freewrite for several minutes about how their memories of their grandmothers are linked to a specific geographical locale and a specific kind of house. I, for example, think of the poor Ridgewood section of Brooklyn, New York and the sound of the "El"–the elevated city trains–repeatedly rattling the windows of my grandparents' cramped apartment as they passed by. North Carolinian grandchildren are likely to summon up visions of more rural or suburban settings for their grandmothers. After sharing our freewrites, I then ask students if they recall such settings in literature, films, or TV shows. *On Golden Pond, Driving Miss Daisy*, and *Golden Girls* come to mind. These activities make students more aware of the North American context in which they read and discuss Allende's (2003) text.

Because ghosts and other supernatural creatures are so much a part of the Allende (2003) family ethos, it is no surprise that they also inhabit this memoir. Characters in her life story, particularly women, sometimes take on powerful, larger-than-life qualities. To her great-grandmother Ester, Allende (2003) ascribes quasi-divine powers that have influenced many of her descendents: "she made judgments on the lives of others; nothing escaped her tiny falcon eyes and her prophet's tongue" (p. 25). Passages like this one should be the subject of close reading by the class. We note the all-seeing, all-knowing qualities of this woman suggested by the phrase "prophet's tongue"; and we see recurring religious diction in the following passage about an aunt of Allende's (2003): "I have a hundred-year-old aunt who aspires to sainthood, and whose only wish has been to go into the convent" (p. 27). The author recounts how this preachy aunt when young "sang religious hymns for hours in her angelic voice" and would loudly denounce the prostitutes on public streets (p. 27). In exalting but also gently satirizing such elderly female relatives, the memoirist blends humor with respect for the spiritual element in their personalities. Is it different from the sometimes-insulting portrayals of elders in our culture? This is a question to pose to students, who usually acknowledge the differences.

In another passage, acknowledging the "esoteric strain" within her family, Allende (2003) describes her great-aunt in clearly mystical terms; she grows a pair of angel's wings: "they were discreet little stumps on her shoulders, erroneously diagnosed by doctors as a bone deformity. Sometimes, depending on where the light was coming from, we could see a halo like a plate of light floating about her head" (p. 59). Allende (2003) notices this great-aunt's angelic serenity and the divine light shining from her—as it does from Agosin's (2000) matriarch Helena. The memoir also pays tribute to the great-aunt as another of Allende's (2003) muses; she hovers over the author as she pursues her creative endeavors: "I have always kept her photograph on my desk so I will recognize her when she slips slyly into the pages of a book or appears in some corner of the house" (p. 59). Are Chileans more comfortable than North Americans with blurring the borders between life and death, between the natural and the supernatural, more inclined toward a magic realism prevalent in Latin American literature, as they portray old women? We consider the cultural and literary construction of old women in Allende's (2003) memoir.

The portrayal of Grandmother Isabel shows us more of this mystical, even superstitious, streak in Chilean culture. Allende (2003) claims that her grandmother—another of Allende's (2003) muses—introduced her to the notion of "multiple dimensions to reality," even before magical realism entered Latin American literary history. This mystical element of their culture is evident in the fact that Chileans nowadays turn to *curanderos* (healers) and are receptive to seers, the horoscope, and even kabbalah. Allende (2003) tells us that Chile has "a delicious oral tradition of evil spirits, interventions of the devil, and dead who rise from their tombs" (p. 64). Then she gives us an example, retelling a tale out of Chiloe (an island fishing community off the south Chilean coast about La Pincoya, "a beautiful damsel who rises from the water to trap unwary men" (p. 65), mentioning also how, "from time immemorial, sailors have deserted their ships, entranced by the longhaired sirens who wait . . . on our beaches" (p. 48). This passage recalls the legend of the demonic ship referred to by Neruda in "Old Women by the Sea." Allende (2003) describes her grandmother as quite comfortable in this otherworldly world.

Allende (2003) herself is confident that Grandmother Isabel will return to visit her family after her death whenever they invite her because she knows well her grandmother's commitment while on earth to contacting the otherworldly world: "she spent her life practicing effects with paranormal phenomena and trying to communicate with the Great Beyond" (p. 66). Her grandmother's magical dimension is evident in her belief "that space is filled with presences, the dead and the living all mixed together" (p. 70). The author clearly subscribes to this "fabulous idea" (p. 70). So Allende (2003) infuses her own portrayals of old family matriarchs with spiritual powers and prophetic wisdom.

Another interesting issue to consider is whether old men are depicted by Allende (2003) in as mystical a manner as old women. In class discussions we examine how the treatment of elderly male relatives in Allende's (2003) book differs from that of females. In her portrait of her grandfather, for example, the author describes his longevity (he lives almost to a hundred) and his mental sharpness: "He lived nearly a century with never a sign of a single loose screw" (p. 32). Through her portrayal of her grandfather, the author denies that senility is inevitable for all elders. She praises her grandfather's clear-eyed intelligence. She also expresses her gratitude that he has educated her by exposing her to the works of Chilean writers (Allende, 2003, p. 111). And she sees him as another of the muses that inspire her to write: "This formidable man gave me the gift of discipline and love for language; without them I could not devote myself to writing today" (Allende, 2003, p. 32). She pays tribute to him for his rationality and keen intellect, so unlike the matriarchs' mystical qualities (Allende, 2003, p. 180).

As to her own senescence, Allende (2003) imagines it with relish and humor as a space to continue her storytelling: "I have tried to polish the details [of my life story] and create my private legend, so that when I am in a nursing home awaiting death I will have something to entertain the other senile old folks with" (p. 180). Even life in a nursing home will be tolerable with stories to tell and hear. The wry humor evident in these fantasies of senescence suggests that Allende (2003) does not really expect senility and does not fear old age–an important lesson for our students that counters the portrayal of dementia in L'Engle's (1974) mother. Allende (2003) is upbeat about elders' position in Chilean, archly noting that Chile is a kissing nation and that therefore the nation shows elders its affection and respect: "older people are kissed mercilessly, even against their will" (p. 101).

Students can clearly expand their understanding of the cultural construction of aging by examining Chile's literature of aging in comparison to their own. Understanding old age leads to greater sympathy for elders and banishes ageist attitudes. If a negative attitude toward the old is culturally constructed, then it can also be culturally deconstructed. Literature can help in the deconstruction. Ultimately this process can bring us to a more conscientious ethic in the treatment of elders within our own society.

In *The Coming of Age*, Simone de Beauvoir (1972) posits that "there is often a very important gap between the myths a society creates and the customs it actually follows" (p. 67). Today ageism exists in the U.S. and may well exist in Chilean society too, even when the traditional stories and contemporary literature teach a respectful conduct toward the old and contain spiritualized portraits of elders. We can fight against ageism by guiding students to the exploration of cross-cultural literary texts that portray elders' humanity and that show readers the spiritual gifts elders can offer to society.

REFERENCES

Adams, A. (1982). *To See You Again*. New York: Knopf.

Agosin, M. (2000). *The Alphabet in My Hands: A Writing Life*. N. A. Hall (Trans.) New Brunswick, NJ & London: Rutgers University Press.

Allende, I. (2003). *My Invented Country: A Nostalgic Journey Through Chile*. M.S. Peden (Trans.) New York: HarperCollins.

Belitt, B. (1996). *Old Women by the Sea* ["Las Viejas del Oceano"]. Selected Poems of Pablo Neruda. New York: Grove Press.

Burke, K. (1989). *Literature as Equipment for Living*. The Critical Tradition: Classic Texts and Contemporary Trends, D. H. Richter (Ed). (pp. 512-517). New York: St. Martin's Press.

Chile: Family Life. Retrieved July 12, 2004 from http://www.settlement.org/cp/english/chile/family.html.

Couve, A. (2003). Seaside Resort. In K. Silver (Ed & Trans.), *Chile: A Traveler's Literary Companion* (pp.85-93). Berkeley, California: Whereabouts Press.

De Beauvoir, S. (1972). *The Coming of Age*. P. O'Brien (Trans.), New York: Putnam's.

De Vos, S. (1998). *Kinship Ties and Solitary Living Among Unmarried Elderly Women: Evidence from Chile and Mexico*. Center for Demography & Ecology, Working Paper No. 98-20. Univ. of Wisconsin-Madison. http://www.ssc.wisc.edu/cde/cdewp/98-20.pdf.

Dorson, R. M. (1967) *Foreword to Folktales of Chile*. Y. Pino-Saavedra & R. Gray (Ed & Trans), Chicago & London: The University of Chicago Press.

Encyclopaedia Judaica. (1972). *Angels*. (Vol. 2, pp. 955-998). Third Printing. Jerusalem: Keter PublishingHouse, Ltd.

Fowler, M., & McCutcheon, P. (1991)(Eds.). *Songs of Experience: An Anthology of Literature on Growing Old*. New York: Ballantine Books

Gullette, M. M. (1997). *Declining to Decline: Cultural Combat and the Politics of the Midlife*. Charlottesville, VA & London: The University Press of Virginia.

Laurence, M. (1993). *The Stone Angel*. Originally published in 1964. Chicago: University of Chicago Press.

L'Engle, M. (1974). *The Summer of the Great-Grandmother*. New York: Farrar, Straus & Giroux.

Lessing, D. (1984). *If the Old Could.... The Diaries of Jane Somers*. New York: Vintage.

Lurie, A. (1998). *The Last Resort: A Novel*. New York: Henry Holt.

Nelson, H. L. (2000). *Stories of my old age*. In M. U. Walker (Ed., p. 75-95). Mother Time: Women, Aging, and Ethics. Lanham, MD; Boulder; New York; Oxford, England: Rowan & Littlefield Publishers, 2000.

Pino-Saavedra, Y. (1967). *Introduction to Folktales of Chile*. In Y. Pino-Saavedra (Ed. & Trans.), Rockwell Gray. Chicago & London: The University of Chicago Press.

Rosenblatt, L. M. (1983). *Literature as Exploration*. Modern Language Association of America. 4th ed.

Schachter-Shalomi, Z., & Miller, R. S. (1995). *From Age-ing to Sage-ing: A Profound New Vision of Growing Older*. New York: Warner Books.

Selden, R. (1989). *A Reader's Guide to Contemporary Literary Theory*. 2nd ed. Lexington, KY: The University Press of Kentucky.

Tresidder, J. (2003). *1001 Symbols: The Illustrated Key to the World of Symbols*. London: Duncan Baird Publishers.

Waxman, B. F. (1997). *To Live in the Center of the Moment: Literary Autobiographies of Aging*. Charlottesville, VA & London: The University Press of Virginia.

Woodward, K. (1991). *Aging and Its Discontents: Freud and Other Fictions*. Bloomington, IN: Indiana University Press.

Woodward, K. (Ed.). *Figuring Age: Women, Bodies, Generations*. Bloomington & Indianapolis: University of Indiana Press.

Gerontology Programs
in Japanese Higher Education:
A Brief History, Current Status,
and Future Prospects

Noriko Tsukada, PhD
Toshio Tatara, PhD

SUMMARY. The development of gerontological education is lagging behind in Japan in spite of Japan's large population of elders. Nevertheless, there
are signs that this may be changing. In this paper we discuss how gerontology
education has evolved in Japan over the past 40 years. Specifically, we provide
an overview of the development of academic societies related to gerontology,
the number of gerontological books published, government statements about
gerontology education, and Japan's only graduate program in gerontology. We
also identify some reasons for the delay in creating gerontology programs and
propose specific steps that might be taken to reverse this trend. *[Article copies
available for a fee from The Haworth Document Delivery Service: 1-800-HAWORTH.*

Noriko Tsukada is Associate Professor, Nihon University Graduate School of Business, 4-8-24 Kudan-Minami, Chiyoda-ku, Tokyo 102-8275, Japan (E-mail: ntsukada@
gsb.nihon-u.ac.jp).
Toshio Tatara is Professor in the Department of Sociology, Shukutoku University,
200 Daiganji-cho, Chuo-ku, Chiba-shi, Chiba-ken 279-0014, Japan.

The authors wish to acknowledge, with appreciation, help in providing them with
literature and information about gerontology education in Japan from Professor Hiroko
Kase of Waseda University (who was on the faculty of Obirin University when the first
draft of this manuscript was prepared) and Mr. Koji Miyauchi of the NLI Research Institute in Tokyo. Their assistance made it possible for the authors to complete this
manuscript.

[Haworth co-indexing entry note]: "Gerontology Programs in Japanese Higher Education: A Brief History,
Current Status, and Future Prospects." Tsukada, Noriko, and Toshio Tatara. Co-published simultaneously in
Gerontology & Geriatrics Education (The Haworth Press, Inc.) Vol. 26, No. 1, 2005, pp. 97-115; and: *Aging
Education in a Global Context* (ed: Dena Shenk, and Lisa Groger) The Haworth Press, Inc., 2005, pp. 97-115.
Single or multiple copies of this article are available for a fee from The Haworth Document Delivery Service
[1-800-HAWORTH, 9:00 a.m. - 5:00 p.m. (EST). E-mail address: docdelivery@haworthpress.com].

E-mail address: <docdelivery@haworthpress.com> Website: <http://www. HaworthPress.com> © 2005 by The Haworth Press, Inc. All rights reserved.]

KEYWORDS. Japan, history of gerontology, gerontology education

The extent of aging in the Japanese population has been marked in recent years due largely to rapidly declining fertility rates on the one hand and extended life expectancies on the other. For example, in 2003 the fertility rate of 1.32 was the lowest ever in Japan, and the proportion of older people in the population was 19.0%. The World Health Organization (WHO) reported that healthy life expectancy in Japan was the highest in the world (WHO, 2000) as was life expectancy at birth ("Nihonjin no Heikin Jumyo," 2003). If the current trends continue, the proportion of older people in the population in this country is expected to reach 26.0% by 2015, when all baby boomers will turn 65 years of age and older.

In view of these demographic changes that are taking place in Japan, the importance of gerontology as an academic discipline for studying and understanding the dynamics and impact of aging is great in this country. It is therefore critical that gerontology education, whereby people would be taught knowledge, skills, and values to appreciate the issues and problems of an aging society and engage in problem-solving efforts, be developed and expanded in Japan. Geriatrics has been a part of the curriculum of Tokyo University's Department of Medicine since 1962, and to date, at least 20 universities across the country have implemented educational programs in geriatrics (Iguchi, Kuzuya, Suzuki, & Umegaki, 1998). As for gerontology education in Japan, very little has been done to date. In this paper we describe the efforts that have taken place to advance gerontological education in this country and review some factors that could possibly help facilitate the expansion of gerontology education in Japan.

THE BIRTH OF GERONTOLOGY AND ITS GROWTH AS AN ACADEMIC DISCIPLINE IN JAPAN

Development of Academic Societies Related to Gerontology

The history of gerontology in Japan began in July 1954 when a small group of medical researchers and social scientists founded an academic organization and named it the Gerontological Association of Japan (GAJ). Over the years, many people wondered why the founders of the GAJ used the term "gerontological" in the English version of the name of the organization, because its Japanese name "Jumyou Gaku Kenkyuu Kai" (a group for the study of life span) could not be directly translated into its English equivalent of "gerontological." However, an examination of the literature published by the GAJ reveals that the founders of the GAJ were aware of the definition of gerontology as the quantitative and qualitative study of the processes of aging and wanted to form an organization of scientists interested in pursuing interdisciplinary research into the phenomena and processes of aging, as suggested by this definition (Watanabe, 1959). Following the formation of the GAJ, their founders maintained that the objective of the association would be to study the phenomena of aging and the factors that would influence the processes of aging, but held that the academic discipline pursuing this objective should be referred to as "Jumyou gaku" (a study of life span) in Japanese (Watanabe, 1959).

The GAJ conducted its first national conference on December 8-9, 1956. This two-day conference, which was referred to as the first Gerontological Congress of Japan, was held at the conference facilities of the Japan Medical Association (JMA) in Tokyo, and nearly 400 people participated in the event (The Gerontological Association of Japan, 1957). The GAJ then consisted of two committees, the Geriatric and the Cultural Sciences Committees. On the first day of the conference, Hiroshige Shiota, the president of the GAJ, delivered a keynote address on "Critical Issues in Gerontology." In his address, Shiota (1957) stressed the importance of "advancing a study of the fundamentals of aging from the perspectives of biology and the medical sciences and of furthering interdisciplinary studies of the social meaning of aging through an integration of various social science disciplines" (p. 6). He further stated that "our measures to combat aging must be developed on the basis of the findings of all these scientific inquiries," and that a new scientific discipline, "gerontology," which was then rapidly becoming known across the world, "should help us with efforts to better understand aging" (Shiota, 1957, p. 6).

The GAJ held its second Gerontological Congress of Japan in Osaka in 1957 and its third in Nagoya in 1958. Judging from how gerontology has evolved in Japan, what happened at the third Congress turned out to be significant. That is, at this Congress, the GAJ changed the name of the Congress to the Gerontological Society of Japan (GSJ), and also renamed their two committees. Thus, the Geriatric Committee became the Japan Geriatric Society (JGS), while the Cultural Sciences Committee was renamed the Japan Socio-Gerontological Society (JSGS) (The Gerontological Association of Japan, 1959). The newly renamed GSJ, along with two component groups, JGS and JSGS, officially began their business in 1959. Subsequently, between 1982 and 2003, four scholarly associations became affiliated with the GSJ as their component group: the Japan Society for Biomedical Gerontology (JSBG) joined the GSJ in 1982; the Japanese Society of Gerodontology (JSG) in 1991; the Japanese Psychogeriatric Society (JPG) in 1999; and the Japan Society of Care Management (JSCM) in 2003. These four groups along with the two original ones still operate within the GSJ today. Although these groups are often referred to as the component groups of the GSJ, each group has its own board of directors who determine the organizational objectives, activity plans, and annual budgets. Each group also has its own constituency and membership. Nevertheless, all of these groups, including the GSJ, share the common goal of advancing scientific studies of aging in Japan. In fact, many members of these groups support an interdisciplinary approach to studying the phenomena and processes of aging and try to practice such an approach through membership in more than one group.

Over the years, all of the groups have grown organizationally by increasing their individual membership. By April 29, 2004 ("The Japan Geriatrics Society," n.d.), the Japan Geriatrics Society had become the largest of all organizations operating within the Gerontological Society of Japan, with 6,400 members, most of whom are geriatricians. The Japanese Psychogeriatric Society is a distant second, with 2,451 members. The Japanese Society of Gerontology is the third largest group, with 1,859 members, the fourth largest one is the Japan Society of Care Management with a reported 1,261 members. Other groups are considerably smaller in terms of their individual membership.

TRENDS IN JAPANESE PUBLICATIONS THAT CONTAIN THE TERMS, "ROUNEN GAKU," "GERONTOLOGY," OR "AGING" IN THE MAIN TITLES OR SUB-TITLES

Over the past 40 years, close to 150 books related to aging have been published in Japan. Figure 1 presents the number of books containing the terms "rounen gaku" (the study of older people), "gerontology," or "aging" in their main titles or sub-titles that were published in Japan between the 1960s and the 2000s. On average, 10 books containing the term "rounen gaku" in their titles or sub-titles were published in each decade, indicating a steady increase in the acceptance of "rounen gaku" mainly among university students and researchers. The popularity of

FIGURE 1. Trends in the publications that contain the terms, "Rounengaku" (Gerontology in Japanese), "Gerontology" or "Aging" in the main titles or sub-titles

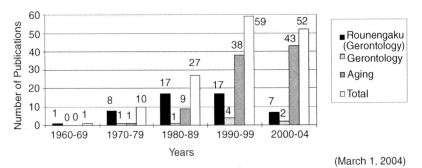

(March 1, 2004)

	1960-69	1970-79	1980-89	1990-99	2000-04
Rounengaku (Gerontology)	1	8	17	17	7
Gerontology	0	1	1	4	2
Aging	0	1	9	38	43
Total	1	10	27	59	52

the English term "aging" in publication titles has risen sharply in the 1990s when a total of 38 books with the term "aging" in their titles or sub-titles were published. Since 2000, a total of 43 books containing the English word "aging" in their titles or sub-titles were published in Japan. It is true that the English term "aging" began to appear frequently in the titles of Japanese books in the early 1990s, when the Japanese government started to strengthen measures to address the effects of aging of the country's population through the Gold Plan and the New Gold Plan. Launched by the Ministry of Health and Welfare in 1989, the Gold Plan set forth Japan's 10 year-plan, with specific numerical objectives, to improve the infrastructures of welfare and health care for older people. It was revised in 1994, and was renamed the New Gold Plan. In contrast, the English word "gerontology" has been used in the publication titles only several times in Japan since the 1960s. This is a little surprising in view of the fact that the word has been well understood by many Japanese researchers and practitioners in the field of aging and that many Japanese have enjoyed membership in the International Gerontological Association (IGA) and the Gerontological Society of

America (GSA) and have regularly participated in the activities of these organizations.

The Term "Rounen Gaku" in Japanese Government Publications

The term "rounen gaku," which means the study of older people, first appeared in a publication of the Japanese Government in 1985, when "Kagaku Gijutsucho Shigen Chosakai" (Resources Study Committee of the Science and Technology Bureau) (1985) issued a report, *"Sukoyakana Shinkoureiki"*(Healthy New Aging). This report predicted that if the aging of the Japanese population continues as fast as it has until now, "by 2020, the proportion of older people in our nation's population will be among the worlds highest" (Kagaku Gijutsucho Shigen Chosakai, 1985, p. 2). Later in the report, the authors stressed that a new academic discipline, "gerontology," would have to be established in Japan to help solve the various problems of an aging society and that the creation of this new discipline would be possible when "such existing academic disciplines as medicine, biology, philosophy, sociology, economics, jurisprudence, psychology, and cultural anthropology that are related to older people are integrated" (Kagaku Gijutsucho Shigen Chosakai, 1985, pp. 75-76).

It took another 12 years until the word "rounen gaku" appeared again in a publication of the Japanese government. In the 1997 edition of a Kousei Hakusho (White Paper), the Ministry of Health and Welfare set up a special column on "rounen gaku" and wrote this comment regarding their expectations for the future of "rounen gaku" in Japan:

> The effects of an aging population upon our society are many and profound. They are also wide-ranging but are related with one another. "Rounen gaku" (gerontology) is an academic discipline that is concerned with the interdisciplinary study of older people and all of the issues faced by an aging society. When we must examine the entire spectrum of an aging society to meet the demands of a new era, the methods of inquiry used by existing disciplines are no longer adequate. Thus, the importance of "rounen gaku" as an academic discipline that would help us understand an aging society has become greatly pronounced. "Rounen gaku" has been developed as an academic discipline in the United States. In the U.S., there have been a large number of educational and research programs on "rounen gaku" at institutions of higher learning. Begin-

ning with an inquiry into the dynamics and processes of aging, the subjects of inquiry in "rounen gaku" are wide-ranging and include, but are not limited to, the psychology of older people, life styles and living conditions of older people, family relationships, social security programs, housing and urban problems, employment and business, and issues of inheritance. In Japan, as we begin to strengthen efforts to understand an aging society, we must learn more about "rounen gaku." (The Ministry of Health and Welfare, 1997, p. 123)

In addition to the term "rounen gaku," the term "karei gaku" (a study of becoming older) has also been used to represent the Japanese equivalent of the English term, "gerontology." When "Tokyoto Seikatsu Bunka Kyoku" (The Tokyo Metropolitan Government's Life and Cultural Affairs Bureau) made its policy recommendations to the government in 2000, there was a reference to "karei gaku" in one of the recommendations regarding aging issues. In that recommendation, this office urged that the perspectives of "karei gaku" (gerontology) be used to examine the issues of an aging society. "Tokyoto Seikatsu Bunka Kyoku"(2000) further stated that a gerontological approach would be more appropriate than approaches of any existing discipline, because "gerontology does not view the phenomenon of aging as a problem and does not see older people as anything unusual" (p. 78). This office also noted that gerontology recognizes aging as a normal process and argued that older people must not be labeled as being special (Tokyoto Seikatsu Bunka Kyoku, 2000, p. 78).

There was another development in gerontology at the national level. That is, in September 2001, Naikakukfu (The Cabinet Office) held a special meeting of policymakers and social policy scholars to discuss the basic assumptions of the nation's strategy for an aging society and stressed the importance of refuting misconceptions (the "mythology for older people," as they were referred to in Japan, with a sarcasm) about older people. The participants agreed that such notions as "older people are unproductive," "older people are not as bright as young people," and "older people are not interested in love or sex" are simply wrong and must be corrected. The meeting organizers were adamant that stereo-typical views of older people are not useful to anyone. They insisted that more scientific studies of older people must be promoted, and concluded that gerontology as a scientific tool to study the process of aging and an aging society would be useful (Naikakufu, 2001, p. 23).

Tokyo Metropolitan Institute of Gerontology (TMIG)

The Tokyo Metropolitan Institute of Gerontology (TMIG) has trained many of the leading Japanese researchers in geriatrics and gerontology over the years. The Institute was founded by the Tokyo Metropolitan Government in 1972 as their research agency in the field of aging. It soon began to assume the role of a national research agency in geriatrics and gerontology by launching research projects of national significance and by collaborating with such organizations as the National Institute on Aging (NIA) in the U.S., the Ukrainian Academy of Medical Sciences in Kiev, and the World Health Organization (WHO). In 1995, the Japanese Government created the National Longevity Research Institute and started to play a more active role in the management of geriatric and gerontological research activities at the national level, but the Institute still remains very active. Today, the Institute is made up of six divisions, namely the divisions on Molecular Gerontology, Neuroscience and Brain Function, Physiology and Aging, Human Science, Cognitive Brain Science, and Basic Research Facilities. Currently it conducts more than 30 research projects, including two long-term projects, "Comprehensive Research on Senile Dementia," which started in 1989, and "Longitudinal Interdisciplinary Study on Aging," which was launched in 1991. Approximately 130 research scientists with a wide range of expertise, and their support personnel, work on these research projects ("Tokyo Metropolitan Institute of Gerontology," n.d.). Some years ago, it was said that the Institute would be one of the three best research institutes in gerontology in the world, along with the earlier-mentioned Ukrainian Academy of Medical Sciences and the National Institute on Aging (NIA) (Karasawa, 1996).

GERONTOLOGY EDUCATION IN JAPAN

Educational Programs on Aging

Yaguchi (1995) reports that many educators in Japan agree that an educational process designed to help reduce prejudice against aging or older people must start early, and to that effect, a special curriculum on aging issues for students between the ages of 6 through 12 was prepared. However, it does not appear that this curriculum on aging has been utilized extensively. In fact, a nation-wide mail survey on the status of aging education, completed by nearly 2,000 elementary and junior high school teachers in the mid-1990s, resulted in findings that were disappointing to many. For example, the survey revealed that, on the whole, teachers themselves held a negative view of older people; only 3.1% of the respondents had received formal training on aging (Takeda, 1995, pp. 83-84). Of the teachers who responded to the survey, only 1.7% had taught material on aging in their classes, and only 1.9% had been actively involved with some type of activities with older people (Takeda, 1995, p. 84). One thing that became clear from this survey was that aging education in primary schools must begin with the teachers.

Gerontology Education at the Undergraduate and Graduate Levels

As of April, 2004, no colleges or universities in Japan offered educational programs leading to the bachelor's degree in gerontology or aging, although classes on gerontology ("rounen gaku," "karei gaku," "aging") are taught at several universities. The following academic departments and universities currently teach gerontology classes: Faculty of Human Development at Kobe University in Kobe; Faculty of Human Life and Environmental Sciences at Ochanomizu University in Tokyo; Department of Human Welfare at Okinawa International University in Naha, Okinawa; and Faculty of Education at Ibaraki University in Mito, Ibaraki. The "rounen gaku" class at Ochanomizu University, which has been taught since 1968 (Sodei, 1995), must be the longest established gerontology course at the university level in Japan. Today, there are 702 four-year universities in Japan, but only four offer courses on gerontology in their undergraduate curricula. This dismal track record in gerontology education at the undergraduate level, however, does not necessarily mean that topics in aging are not taught in Japanese universities. According to the Japanese Association of Schools of Social Work (JASSW), an organization similar to the Council on Social Work Education (CSWE) in the U.S., a total of 176 four-year universities and junior colleges are currently approved by the Ministry of Education and Science to offer Bachelor's or Associate degrees in Social Work. Given that inclusion of the courses on "social welfare for older people" and "field practicum in aging" in the social work curricula is required by the Government, these 176 member universities of JASSW all provide their social work majors with a considerable amount of education in aging.

At the graduate level, Obirin University Graduate School of International Studies in Tokyo is the only institution of higher learning in Japan that currently offers a Master's degree program in gerontology. Effective April 2004, this graduate school became the nation's first institution that administers a doctoral program in gerontology. In addition to these graduate gerontology programs at Obirin, the other graduate schools or departments across the country that offer classes on gerontology are the Graduate School of Cultural Studies and Human Science at Kobe University in Kobe; Graduate School of Humanities and Sciences at Ochanomizu University in Tokyo; Graduate School of Regional Cultures at Okinawa International University in Naha, Okinawa; Graduate School of Human Sciences at Waseda University in Tokyo; and Nihon University Graduate School of Business in Tokyo. It is noticeable that many of these gerontology classes are more advanced than those that are taught at the undergraduate level, and some of them (e.g., educational gerontology, socio-gerontology) could be defined as applied-gerontology classes. There are a total of 529 graduate schools and programs in Japan, but only five provide classes in gerontology, as described above. In contrast to the U.S., Japan puts more emphasis on social work education at the undergraduate level than at the graduate level, and as a result, there are only 47 graduate programs in social work in the country. These programs all must offer courses on "social welfare of older people," "welfare laws for the aged," or something similar, as required by the Government.

GERONTOLOGY PROGRAM AT OBIRIN UNIVERSITY GRADUATE SCHOOL OF INTERNATIONAL STUDIES

About Obirin University

Obirin University, founded in 1966 by Yasuzo Shimizu, a Christian missionary, is located in Machida city (pop. 400,000) about 20 miles southwest of Tokyo. The university aims to provide young people with a liberal arts education, and is part of Obirin Gakuen, a large educational institution that includes a kindergarten, a junior high school, a senior high school, a junior college, and a graduate school, in addition to the university. Today, approximately 9,300 students (of whom 7,000 are in the university) attend various schools of the institution. Obirin University is composed of the undergraduate colleges of the Humanities, Economics, International Studies, Business and Public Administration, as well as a Graduate School of International Studies. The nation's first graduate program in gerontology is housed within this graduate school.

The Obirin Graduate School of International Studies started in 1993 when it opened with two Master's degree programs, one in International Relations and the other in Pan-Pacific Cultural Studies. After it was shown that these two programs were a success, Master's programs in Higher Education Administration and Foreign Language Instruction were added in 2001. Subsequently, two other Master's programs, one in Human Science and the other in Gerontology, were created in 2002, bringing the total number of Master's programs to six. The Ministry of Education, Culture, Sports, Science and Technology capped the total number of students who may enroll in these six programs at 320 at any given time. In addition to these Master's programs, the Graduate School also offers three small doctoral programs, including one in gerontology.

Because students pursuing graduate degrees in Higher Education Administration, Foreign Language Instruction, and Gerontology focus mainly on returning or non-traditional students who may already be employed, the Administration of Obirin University decided to offer evening and weekend classes at a location that would be easily accessible via public transportation from the center of Tokyo ("Obirin Shinjyuku," n.d.). This approach of making graduate programs more accessible to non-traditional students has also been implemented by other universities in recent years, and several of them have set up classrooms in office buildings in the center of Tokyo and begun operating evening and weekend classes. Some even hold classes on Sundays.

Gerontology at the Obirin Graduate School of International Studies

The gerontology Master's program at the Obirin Graduate School of International Studies was first offered in April 2002, with the main purpose of "educating future professionals who would be equipped with knowledge and skills to effectively engage in problem-solving activities in an aging society" ("Obirin Nihon," n.d.). The educational and research objectives of this two-year graduate program are three-fold: (1) to help improve the quality of life of older people; (2) to promote greater social contributions by older people; and (3) to help strengthen intergenerational exchanges of ideas and activities (see Table 1). In Japan, all educational institutions, including colleges and universities, must receive formal approval from the Ministry of Education and Science for any academic degrees they confer and for the respective requirements. To receive the Master's in Gerontology, students must complete the required coursework, write a Master's thesis, and pass written final examinations in a period of two years. There is no requirement for students to complete an agency-based practicum, but students must take a supervised research course in which they learn research methods in gerontology. Non-traditional students who are employed may choose to write a research paper based on some aspects of their job-related activities instead of a more scholarly master's thesis.

The rules of the Ministry of Education, Culture, Sports, Science and Technology require that, with some exceptions, students seeking a master's degree in Japan complete a minimum of 30 "tan i" (academic credit units) in two years. Each course is worth 2 "tan i" and usually meets

TABLE 1. Curriculum for Master's Program in Gerontology

		Subjects	Credit Units
Master's in Gerontology	Core Courses	Gerontology	2
		Geriatrics I	2
		Geriatrics II	2
		Geriatric Psychology I	2
		Geriatric Psychology II	2
		Gerontological Social Work	2
		Sociology of Aging	2
	Specialized Courses	Health Promotion of Aging I	2
		Health Promotion of Aging II	2
		Geriatric Nursing Care	2
		Death Education	2
		Aging Policies	2
		Psychology of Reminiscing I	2
		Psychology of Reminiscing II	2
		Gerontological Research Method I	2
		Gerontological Research Method II	2
		Social Statistics	2
		Geriatric Rehabilitation	2
		Practice in Gerontology I	2
		Practice in Gerontology II	2
	Seminars	Master's thesis I (one year around)	2
		Master's thesis II (one year around)	2

once a week for 90 minutes 12 or 13 weeks per semester. To graduate, therefore, students in Obirin's Gerontology Master's program must successfully complete at least 15 different courses. Additionally, students must take the supervised research course, which is worth 4 "tan i" in total.

As of April, 2004, Obirin's graduate program in gerontology had 12 faculty members of whom four professors and one associate professor hold full-time tenured positions; the seven others hold part-time positions. All full-time faculty members hold doctorates (four MDs and one PhD) and have extensive research experience in Japan and abroad. They have also published widely in their fields which include geriatrics, gerontology, psychology, geriatric psychology, developmental psychology, epidemiology, public health, and hygiene. Four of the five full-time faculty members were at one time senior researchers at the Tokyo Metropolitan Institute of Gerontology (TMIG).

Except for one person who is a senior researcher at the Tokyo Metropolitan Institute of Gerontology, the part-time faculty members are all tenured faculty members of other universities. They are well known in their research communities which include geriatric psychology, developmental psychology, geriatric nursing, gerontology, rehabilitation science, occupational therapy, labor relations, social policy, and social welfare. The qualifications and teaching assignments of these faculty members had to be reviewed and approved by the Ministry of Education, Culture, Sports, Science and Technology when the graduate program in gerontology was created and approved. All applicants to graduate programs in Japan have to take an entrance examination. The entrance examination to Obirin's graduate program in gerontology consists of an English test, a short essay on the applicant's research plan, and a face-to-face interview. Students returning from abroad and other applicants who hold government-issued certificates for English proficiency may be exempt from taking the English test. Obirin's graduate program in gerontology is competitive in that each year there are more applicants than the number of students the program can accept, which is 20 students a year.

The graduate students in gerontology at Obirin are very diverse in terms of their backgrounds. For example, of one recent graduating class, nearly one-half were nurses, the others were retirees, social workers, office workers, part-time workers, persons looking for employment or a career change, recent college graduates, and housewives. The ages of the students in this class ranged from 24 to 72, while the ratio of female to male students was close to 1:1. The nation's only doctoral program in gerontology at Obirin University, which started in April 2004, accepted seven students.

Four of these students are graduates of Obirin's Master's program in gerontology, while the remaining three came from other universities. Most are licensed in clinical psychology, occupational therapy, physical therapy, or nursing, but have expressed an interest in seeking university faculty positions after completing their doctoral dissertations.

ISSUES IN GERONTOLOGY EDUCATION IN JAPAN AND FUTURE PROSPECTS

The International Longevity Center-Japan issued a report, "*Nihon ni okeru Rounengaku Kyoiku Kouza Kaisetsu no tameno Yobi Chosa Kenkyu Houkokusho*" (Pre-investigation of development of Gerontology education in Japan), in 1995, and in the preface of this report, Ibe (1995), then the president of the Center, stressed an urgent need for starting gerontology programs at graduate schools across the country. In the same report, Sasaki (1995) argued that a gerontological approach should be much broader than just being concerned with the integration of any two academic disciplines. He went on to mention two reasons for why ideas in gerontology developed abroad would not be accepted in Japan if they were brought into the country without being modified. First, these ideas would not be useful in Japan because they were developed in countries where the extent of aging in the populations was not as great as it is in Japan. Second, Japanese policies, practices, and circumstances dealing with an aging society were so unique that they could not be easily explained or understood by theories that were developed in other countries. Sasaki (1995) therefore proposed the creation of a graduate program in Japan that would teach macro-level social policy and Japan's own brand of gerontology (p. 3).

Additionally, Shibata (2000), who is currently on Obirin's graduate faculty in gerontology and who had been involved with efforts to found Obirin's graduate program, warned in one of the International Longevity Center-Japan publications that any delay in getting gerontology firmly accepted as an academic discipline and as an applied profession in Japan would delay the elimination of ageism and the establishment of social policy that would help improve the quality of life of elders and their opportunities for making social contributions. He then urged policymakers and professionals to continue their efforts to disseminate gerontology in Japan, and he introduced the idea of creating a national gerontology center which would serve as the basis for all efforts to promote gerontology, with financial and political support from the corporate, governmental, academic, and civic sectors (Shibata, 2000, p. 5).

Starting with the formation of the Gerontological Association of Japan (GAJ) in 1954, there has been considerable effort to establish educational programs in gerontology. Along the way, these efforts were not without support from the government, and academic and research communities, as mentioned earlier. Particularly, the Ministry of Health, Labour and Welfare has lately intensified its support for the recognition of gerontology as a method for understanding the issues of an aging society. In the research community, there has been a marked increase in recent years in the number of Japanese researchers attending and making presentations at conferences of such organizations as the Gerontological Society of America (GSA) and the International Gerontological Association (IGA). Some of these researchers earned graduate degrees from gerontology programs abroad and are involved with gerontology education in Japan. Yet, Obirin's graduate program in gerontology and a dozen or so of under-graduate and graduate classes on gerontology are the only educational programs in gerontology that exist in Japan today. What accounts for this rather lean outcome of all the efforts to get a gerontology education established in Japan?

POSSIBLE REASONS FOR THE SLOW PROGRESS IN GERONTOLOGY EDUCATION IN JAPAN

First, although the Ministry of Education, Culture, Sports, Science and Technology has somewhat relaxed its control, it still controls almost every aspect of education in Japan. For example, without the Ministry's formal permission, universities cannot even change the name of an academic department; much less start a new degree program. This makes it impossible for any new educational program to be initiated without being decreed by law (Tsukada, 2001). The Ministry of Education, Culture, Sports, Science and Technology has not yet shown its active support for gerontology education. Second, it is true that the Ministry of Health, Labour and Welfare has officially stated in several of its publications that gerontology would be a useful academic discipline in an aging society and has supported efforts to promote educational programs in gerontology, as described earlier. However, this national agency has no jurisdiction over matters in formal education and cannot act officially on behalf of those who try to establish educational programs in gerontology across the country.

Third, although there are several national associations in Japan that represent the interests of researchers and practitioners in the field of aging, none of them is like the Association for Gerontology in Higher Education (AGHE), which was created for the specific purpose of promoting and advancing educational programs in gerontology in U.S. colleges and universities (Takahashi, 2000; Tsukada, 2001). In other words, there are currently no organizations in Japan that are specifically designed to promote gerontology education. Fourth, it has been suggested that Japanese translations of theoretical materials in gerontology created in other countries are often vague and confusing to Japanese educators (Miyajima, 1995). Shibata (1995) argued that for these reasons, gerontology has not yet been established as an academic discipline as firmly as has geriatrics. In light of this situation, officials of the Ministry of Education, Culture, Sports, Science and Technology are not likely to become enthused about promoting formal gerontology education in Japan anytime soon.

RECOMMENDATIONS

What, then, would be the best way to overcome all of these obstacles to advancing gerontology in Japan? Clearly, we must take small but realistic and well-calculated steps to move forward by taking advantage of what we now have in terms of expertise and resources in gerontology or aging studies. First, we have to strengthen our existing associations of gerontological researchers in Japan by increasing their active membership and by promoting greater opportunities for their research. In this respect, we must aggressively seek greater support from private foundations and corporate communities in the form of grants and contracts. Second, we must encourage and support university students interested in gerontology to go abroad for graduate study in gerontology. As we are faced with the problems of an aging society in Japan, it is imperative that we rely on the expertise of those who have the knowledge and skills in solving these problems. It is clear that Japan's need for the expertise of gerontologists will continue to grow, but our country is not yet serious about formally training gerontologists. Third, we have to expand educational programs in aging at both the undergraduate and graduate levels and become actively involved in teaching and research in the field of aging. Although courses on aging are being taught in a number of colleges and universities in a variety of departments, Obirin is currently the only institution of higher learning in Japan that offers graduate programs in gerontology. Thus, the chances for any gerontologist to be able to teach a formal gerontology course in a Japanese university is very slim. However, faculty could make efforts to become involved in teaching university-level aging courses in such disciplines as nursing, social work, and clinical psychology. Fourth, by being involved with civic and social activities at the community level, those of us who are trained in gerontology must become active advocates for disseminating knowledge about the nature of aging and an aging society. All practicing gerontologists must make it their personal responsibility to speak about the importance of creating gerontology programs at colleges and universities across the country.

CONCLUSIONS

As shown in this paper, the fact remains that currently there is only one Master's program in gerontology in Japan, and this program generates about two dozens of trained gerontologists each year. In addition, Obirin University, which operates this program, started a small doctoral program in gerontology in April 2004, with an enrollment of seven students. Even if all goes well, the first gerontologist with a doctorate earned in Japan would not graduate before 2008 or 2009 at the earliest. A handful of undergraduate and graduate programs that offer courses in gerontology are unlikely to start providing academic degrees in gerontology. It is indeed regrettable that the growth of gerontology education in institutions of higher learning is lagging so far behind in Japan, in spite of the fact that Japan has one of the oldest populations in the world. We firmly stand by what we stated in the recommendations, and we believe that we as researchers and practitioners in gerontology can make progress in gerontology graduate education if we keep plugging away at the specifics tasks we outlined above. We are not sure if our government will do anything spectacular to promote gerontology education in our country, but we are certain that if we are not going to make efforts to help ourselves in this endeavor, no one else will help us to create gerontology education in Japan.

REFERENCES

Ibe, H. (1995). Hashigaki [Introduction]. *Nihon ni okeru rounengaku kyoiku kouza kaisetsu no tameno yobi chosa kenkyu houkokusho* [Pre-investigation of development of gerontology education in Japan]. March, 1995. International Longevity Center-Japan. Tokyo, Japan.

Iguchi, A., Kuzuya, M., Suzuki, Y., & Umegaki, H. (1998). Rounenigaku kyoiku [Geriatric Education], *Journal of Geriatric Medicine, 35*, 867-872.

Kagaku Gijutsucho Shigen Chosakai [Resources Study Committee of the Science and Technology Bureau] (1985)(ed.). *Sukoyakana shinkoureiki: Rouka boushi to koureiki no shakaitekio ni kansuru chousa houkoku* [Healthy new aging: Findings of a study of the prevention of aging and social adjustment in old age]. Tokyo, Japan.

Karasawa, A. (1996).Tokyo Metropolitan Research Institute. In *Gendai Aging Jiten* [New Encyclopedia of Aging], p. 339. Waseda University. Tokyo, Japan.

Miyajima, H. (1995). Koreishakai no shakai keizaiteki shomondai: Rounengaku ni nozomu mono [Economic problems in an aging society in Japan: Implications for Gerontology]. *Nihon ni okeru rounengaku kyoiku kouza kaisetsu no tameno yobi chosa kenkyu houkokusho* [Pre-investigation of development of gerontology education in Japan]. March, 1995. International Longevity Center-Japan. Tokyo, Japan.

Naikakufu [The Cabinet Office](2001). *Kourei shakai taisaku no suishin no kihonteki arikata ni tsuite–Nenrei kara jiyuu na shakai wo mezashite* [Basic strategies for an aging society–Toward an age-free society]. September, 2001. Tokyo, Japan.

Nihonjin no heikin jumyo [Life expectancy of Japanese people]. (2003, July 12) Nihon Keizai Newspaper, p. 1.

Obirin Nihon hatsu: Rounengaku no kyoiku kenkyu (n.d.) [Japan's first gerontological education program]. Retrieved April 30, 2004, from Obirin University Web site: http://www.obirin.ac.jp/graduateschool/300/315.html

Obirin Shinjuku campus no jugyo (n.d.) [Lectures at Shinjuku Campus]. Retrieved May 1, 2004, from Obirin University Web site: http://www.obirin.ac.jp/graduateschool/330/303r.html

Sasaki, T. (1995). Souron [An overview]. *Nihon ni okeru rounengaku kyoiku kouza kaisetsu no tameno yobi chousa kenkyu houkokusho* [Pre-investigation of development of gerontology education in Japan], pp.1-3. March, 1995. International Longevity Center-Japan. Tokyo, Japan.

Shibata, H. (1995). Kenkougaku, igakumen kara mita roujin [Older people from aspects of health and medical sciences]. *Nihon ni okeru rounengaku kyoiku kouza kaisetsu no tameno yobi chousa kenkyu houkokusho* [Pre-investigation of development of gerontology education in Japan], pp. 12-19. March, 1995. International Longevity Center-Japan. Tokyo, Japan.

Shibata, H. (2000). Nihon ni okeru Gerontology no kakuritsu wo mezashite [Toward development of Gerontology]. *Nihon ni okeru Gerontology no kakuritsu ni kansuru kenkyu houkokusho* [Report on development of gerontology in Japan]. International Longevity Center-Japan, pp. 1-8. Tokyo, Japan.

Shiota, H.(1957). Gerontology no motsu kadai [Critical issues in Gerontology]. *The Second Annual Report of Gerontological Association of Japan*, p. 6. Tokyo, Japan.

Sodei, T. (1995). Nihon ni okeru Rounengaku kouza no shoukai-Ochanomizu joshi daigaku no case wo chuushin ni [Introduction of Gerontology in Japan: Case of Ochanomizu University]. *Nihon ni okeru rounengaku kyoiku kouza kaisetsu no tameno yobi chousa kenkyu houkokusho* [Pre-investigation of development of gerontology education in Japan]. International Longevity Center-Japan, pp. 4-11. Tokyo, Japan.

Takahashi, R. (2000). America ni okeru koutou kyoiku: Gerontology kyoukai no katsudou to nihon ni okeru kongo no kadai [Activities of AGHE in the U.S. and challenges in Japan]. *Nihon ni okeru Gerontology no kakuritsu ni kansuru kenkyu houkokusho* [Report on development of Gerontology in Japan]. International Longevity Center-Japan, pp. 9-16. Tokyo, Japan.

Takeda, K. (1995). Kyoushi no koureisha image [Images of teachers toward older people]. *Chiiki shakai ni okeru koureisha ni kansuru fukushi kyoiku no genjo ni tsuite no chousa houkokusho* [A report of the current status of social welfare education concerning older people in the local communities]. International Longevity Center-Japan, pp. 70-84. Tokyo, Japan.

The Gerontological Association of Japan (1957). Chogen [Introduction]. *The Second Annual Reports of the Association of Japan*, p. 1. Tokyo, Japan.

The Gerontological Association of Japan (1959). Nihon rounen gakkai no hossoku [Birth of Gerontological Society of Japan]. *The Third Annual Reports of the Gerontological Association of Japan*, pp. 259-262. Tokyo, Japan.

The Japan Geriatrics Society (n.d.). Retrieved February 25, 2004, from http://www.jpn-geriat-soc.or.jp/kanren/dantai.html

The Ministry of Health and Welfare (1997). *Kousei Hakusho* [White Paper], p. 123. Tokyo, Japan.

Tokyo Metropolitan Institute of Gerontology (n.d.). Retrieved June 6, 2003, from http://www.tmig.or.jp

Tokyoto Seikatsu Bunka Kyoku [The Tokyo Metropolitan Government's Life and Cultural Affairs Bureau] (2000). *Tokyoto shohi seikatsu taisaku shingikai toushin* [Policy recommendations of Tokyo Metropolitan Government's Consumer Life Policy Council]. December, 2000. Tokyo, Japan.

Tsukada, N. (2001). Rounengaku no shiten kara mita koureisha gyakutai [Elder abuse: A gerontological viewpoint]. In T. Tatara (Ed.), *Koureisha Gyakutai–Nihon no genjou to kadai* [Elder abuse: Current status and issues in Japan](pp. 153-177). Chuuou Houki, September, 2001. Tokyo, Japan.

Watanabe, S. (1959). Nihon no Gerontology no Houkou [Future direction of Gerontology in Japan], *The Third Annual Reports of the Gerontological Association of Japan*, pp. 1-6. Tokyo, Japan.

WHO (2000). The World Health Report 2000-Health Systems: Improving Performance, World Health Organization, p. 176.

Yaguchi, K. (1995). Koureisha ni kansuru fukushi kyoiku [Education in welfare for older people]. *Chiiki shakai ni okeru koureisha ni kansuru fukushi kyouiku no genjo ni tsuiteno chousa kenkyu houkokusho* [A report of the current status of social welfare education concerning older people in the local communities]. International Longevity Center-Japan, pp. 1-17. Tokyo, Japan.

Gerontology Education and Research in Kenya: Establishing a U.S.-African Partnership in Aging

Sharon V. King, PhD
Mugo Gachuhi, PhD
Gillian Ice, PhD
Maria Cattell, PhD
Frank Whittington, PhD

SUMMARY. This article reprises four presentations on "Gerontology Education in Kenya," a seminar at the 2004 Annual Meeting of the Asso-

Sharon King is Assistant Research Professor, Gerontology Institute, Georgia State University, P.O. Box 3984, Atlanta, GA 30302-3984 (E-mail: gersvk@langate.gsu.edu).

Mugo Gachuhi is Coordinator of Gerontology Programs, Department of Sociology, Kenyatta University, Nairobi, Kenya.

Gillian Ice is Assistant Professor, Department of Social Medicine, Ohio University College of Osteopathic Medicine, Athens, OH.

Maria Cattell is a Research Associate, Field Museum of Natural History, Chicago, IL.

Frank Whittington is Director, Gerontology Institute, Georgia State University, Atlanta, GA.

The authors wish to thank Professor Everett M. Standa, Vice Chancellor, Kenyatta University; Professor Jude Ongong'a, Deputy Vice Chancellor for Academics, Kenyatta University; Dr. Charles Ngome, Director of the Kenyatta University Bureau of Educational Research; Professor Paul Achola, Chair, Department of Sociology, Kenyatta University; and John Hicks, Assistant Provost for International Affairs, Georgia State University, without whose help the collaboration between Georgia State University and Kenyatta University would not have been possible.

[Haworth co-indexing entry note]: "Gerontology Education and Research in Kenya: Establishing a U.S.-African Partnership in Aging." King, Sharon V. et al. Co-published simultaneously in *Gerontology & Geriatrics Education* (The Haworth Press, Inc.) Vol. 26, No. 1, 2005, pp. 117-135; and: *Aging Education in a Global Context* (ed: Dena Shenk, and Lisa Groger) The Haworth Press, Inc., 2005, pp. 117-135. Single or multiple copies of this article are available for a fee from The Haworth Document Delivery Service [1-800-HAWORTH, 9:00 a.m. - 5:00 p.m. (EST). E-mail address: docdelivery@haworthpress.com].

ciation of Gerontology in Higher Education. It describes the process by which the Gerontology Institute of Georgia State University established a 3-year gerontology education and research partnership with Kenyatta University in Nairobi, Kenya, and the field experiences of two scholars who have conducted aging research in Kenya. We provide four key elements of cultural competence and recommendations for American gerontologists wishing to establish international linkages. *[Article copies available for a fee from The Haworth Document Delivery Service: 1-800-HAWORTH. E-mail address: <docdelivery@haworthpress.com> Website: <http://www.HaworthPress.com> © 2005 by The Haworth Press, Inc. All rights reserved.]*

KEYWORDS. Africa, gerontology, education

During the past decade, the term "global aging" has become common *parlance* both within and outside the field of gerontology. The demographic realities of the aging world population, with its social, economic, and political implications, have finally attracted the attention of world leaders and policy-makers, as well as professionals in the field of aging. Since 1990, two World Assemblies on Aging have convened, with the third in progress in Mexico, as we write this article. In the United States, the International Day of Older Persons is now an official national event, and an increasing number of aging advocacy and service organizations have established programs or divisions dedicated to international aging issues, such as AARP's "Global Aging Program" and the Gerontological Society of America's "Global Connections." In 2004, five gerontologists with an interest in aging in Africa–Drs. Sharon King and Frank Whittington of the Gerontology Institute of Georgia State University; Dr. Mugo Gachuhi, a faculty member of the Kenyatta University Bureau of Educational Research in Nairobi, Kenya; Dr. Maria Cattell, an anthropologist and Research Associate with the Field Museum of Natural History in Chicago; and Dr. Gillian Ice, Assistant Professor of Biological Anthropology and Gerontology at Ohio University College of Osteopathic Medicine and immediate past president of the Association for Gerontology and Anthropology (AAGE)–teamed up for a seminar on "Establishing Gerontology Education in Kenya" at the 2004 annual meeting of the Association for Gerontology in Higher Education (AGHE). In this article, we recount our AGHE presentations and provide an overview of the process that led to the Kenyatta University/ Georgia State University gerontology education and research partnership. In addition, we discuss the educational implications and cultural competence issues of gerontological research in Kenya and offer some considerations for gerontology educators and students interested in African aging.

BACKGROUND

The Global Focus on Aging

The interest in global aging among U.S. scholars has been fueled, in part, by the growing number of foreign-born elders in America. Although elderly immigrants comprise only 8.75 percent of the total U.S. elderly population (Angel, 2003), some demographic forecasts show the current aged immigrant population will increase from 2.8 million to 4.5 million by 2010 (Angel, 2003). Further, older immigrants are augmenting the overall number of older ethnic Americans, which is projected to be 15% of the total elderly population by 2025 (Barresi & Stull, 1993).

As opportunities to study aging among foreign-born and ethnic American elders increase, many U.S. gerontologists are gaining an awareness of international aging issues and are participating in international gerontology meetings, such as the Second World Assembly on Aging in Madrid in 2002. The World Assembly on Aging has created a networking forum for gerontologists worldwide and has focused attention on the challenges faced by older adults in developing countries. At the 2002 Madrid World Assembly, United Nations Secretary General Kofi Annan mentioned three challenges of aging in developing countries: (1) the marginalization of older adults who lose traditional family support and social networks as people move to the cities, (2) the HIV/AIDS crisis that is forcing many older adults to care for orphaned children, and (3) the deterioration of the social security and health systems in support of older adults in developing countries (Fenech, 2002).

AGING IN AFRICA

Many African countries face all three of these challenges, as their older populations grow. The demographics of African aging have fostered greater attention to older persons' needs among scholars, service workers, and policy-makers. Nana Apt, Dean of Academic Affairs at Ashesi University in Ghana and current director of the African

Gerontological Society, points to Africa's "cultural revolution"–the so-cial, economic, and political changes that have occurred since the end of co-lonialism–as one of the motivations for the growing interest in African aging. She argues that it is important "to analyze the position of older persons in the absence of the traditional social structural systems, if we are to devise alternative ways that would better accommodate them in the new order of cultural reforms" (Apt, 2002a, p. x). Monica Ferreira, director of the The Albertina and Walter Sisulu Institute of Ageing in Africa at the University of Cape Town and a pioneer in African geron-tology, notes that only recently have African elders had the opportunity, through participation in research studies, to articulate their own experi-ences (Ferreira, 1999). From a research perspective, investigations of the aging experience in Africa can provide important base-line data for aging research among ethnic minorities of African descent in other countries, including the United States (Makoni & Stroeken, 2002).

Some topics about African aging that have attracted the attention of scholars in recent years include: changes in traditional living arrange-ments and family relationships (Mba, 2003; Bongaarts & Zimmer, 2002; Apt, 2002b); the impact of HIV/AIDS on older adults (Wilson & Adamchak, 2001; International HIV/AIDS Alliance & HelpAge Inter-national, 2003; Eke, 2003; Akinsola, 2000); ageism and elder abuse (Van der Geest, 2002; Gorman, 2000; Joubert & Lindgren, 2003); the impact of poverty on aging (Williams, 2003; Adamchak, 1996); aging policy (Bailey & Turner, 2002; Ferreira, 2000; Lloyd, 2002); and men-tal health and aging (Ineichen, 2000; Ferreira & Makoni, 1999; 2002).

Aging Advocacy in Kenya

In Kenya, the number of people over 60 years is estimated to be about 1.1 million, forming 4% of the total population. This figure is projected to increase by 117% by the year 2030 (Kinsella & Velkoff, 2001). In his proposal to the chair of the Kenyatta University sociology department for the development of a gerontology curriculum, Dr. Mugo Gachuhi emphasized the importance of equipping Kenyan educators, students, service providers, and policy-makers with the gerontological educa-tion and skills necessary to meet the needs of a rapidly aging popula-tion. In addition to the aging of the Kenyan population, Dr. Gachuhi stated two additional reasons for the need to train Kenyatta University students, faculty, and service providers in gerontology: (1) the lack of extensive research, including socioeconomic and quality of life studies, on Kenya's older population, and (2) a lack of national preparedness for the implementation of aging-related policies and programs.

Dr. Gachuhi's advocacy efforts have helped place Kenyatta University at the forefront of the aging movement in Kenya, as the university seeks to establish the study of aging as both an academic discipline and an area of public policy development. As a teacher-training institution, Kenyatta University is an ideal setting for a program in gerontology education. Situated about 18 kilometers from Nairobi, Kenyatta University was established as an educational institution in 1965, when the British Government handed over the Templer Barracks to the Kenya Government. These were converted into an institution of higher learning known as Kenyatta College. Following the Act of Parliament of 1970, Kenyatta College became a constituent College of the University of Nairobi, admitting its first 200 students in 1972, and is the only Kenyan institution of higher learning training teachers at both undergraduate and postgraduate levels. University status was achieved in 1985. Kenyatta University currently offers five undergraduate degrees (Bachelor of Arts, Bachelor of Commerce, Bachelor of Education, Bachelor of Science, and Bachelor of Environmental Studies) and six graduate degrees (master's and doctoral) in social science, science, education, environmental science, music, public health and environment, and home economics.

Kenyatta University's plans to establish a gerontology training program prompted Dr. Gachuhi to network with gerontologists in the U.S. and eventually led to the establishment of a partnership between his university and the Georgia State University Gerontology Institute. This partnership networked both institutions with other U.S. scholars conducting aging research in Kenya, including Maria Cattell, who has conducted research among aging families in Kenya for over 20 years, and Dr. Gillian Ice, who currently conducts stress research among older members of the Luo community in western Kenya.

ESTABLISHING A GERONTOLOGY EDUCATION PARTNERSHIP IN AFRICA

Following their first visit to Kenyatta University, Frank Whittington and Sharon King of the Georgia State University (GSU) Gerontology Institute heard a recurring query from their GSU colleagues and others: "How did you get connected to Africa?" The simple truth is we can take little credit for the initiation of our international partnership. Our involvement in aging in Africa was the result of Dr. Gachuhi's search for an American gerontology program that would be willing to partner with Kenyatta University (KU) in the development of a gerontology curriculum that would demonstrate both the appropriateness and practicality of an aging focus in higher education in Kenya. Dr. Gachuhi contacted Mary MacKinnon, the GSU Institute's Director of Student Affairs who coordinates the gerontology certificate program, to inquire about the certificate curriculum. Ms. MacKinnon arranged a meeting with the Institute staff for Dr. Gachuhi, who was visiting family members in Atlanta in June, 2002. During his visit, Dr. Gachuhi stated that his university "would be grateful" if GSU would be in a position to assist KU in its efforts to "offer a gerontology diploma to students and offer short-term courses to service providers from the communities and organizations in the country dealing with older persons and aging" (Gachuhi, 2004).

When we first met Dr. Gachuhi, we anticipated only a cordial networking visit with a fellow-gerontologist from another country. After the meeting, it was clear that we had met a *comrade in arms* in the crusade to advance the study of aging. By the end of the conversation, all parties recognized the potential benefit of a partnership, but we were not sure how to make such a partnership a reality. Clearly, travel to Kenya was necessary to meet with the administration and faculty at Kenyatta University; however, like most gerontology programs, the GSU Institute's budget was limited and included no international travel funds.

From that point, a series of serendipitous events cleared the path for GSU and KU to establish a gerontology partnership. The GSU Office of International Affairs provides seed grants, through the International Strategic Initiatives program (ISI), to establish links with institutions in other countries that could lead to more substantial external funding. We wrote a proposal and received a $5,000 ISI grant to cover the costs of travel and other program expenses for the establishment of a link with Kenyatta University. The successful proposal included a rationale for the partnership, based on the aging of the Kenyan population and the impending demand for professionals trained in the field of aging. The proposal listed two main goals for the partnership: (1) to plan and implement a curriculum for a gerontology certificate program at Kenyatta University, and (2) to develop collaborative aging research projects. The specific aims of the proposal were: (1) to provide faculty development in gerontology education, (2) to help KU faculty design an interdisciplinary curriculum in gerontology, and (3) to create a collaborative research plan to expand both institutions' capacity for the study of ethnicity and aging.

During our initial 8-day trip to Nairobi in February, 2003, we worked with Dr. Gachuhi and other KU faculty to develop a Memorandum of Understanding between GSU and KU, based on the stated objectives of the proposal. We presented an overview of GSU's gerontology education and research program at a seminar for Kenyan aging advocates and government social service administrators and explored mutual research interests with KU faculty. We also spent time in the field observing a home for the aged and a day center for older adults in the Kibera community, one of the largest slums in Africa. What would prove to be a very important meeting was arranged for the GSU team by the KU Bureau of Educational Research with HelpAge Kenya, a non-governmental organization (NGO) dedicated to the well-being of older people in Kenya and a founding member of HelpAge International, a 52-country NGO, which has its African regional office in Nairobi.

Now completing its 2nd year, the KU-GSU partnership is moving forward on its projected course. In August, 2003, the Gerontology Institute received a second ISI seed grant which provided travel funds for two additional visits to Kenya. During a visit in May, 2004, Sharon King presented an introduction to gerontology mini-course as in-service training for KU faculty. Also, in keeping with the goals of the ISI grant, GSU and KU are collaborating on two grant proposals: one for an intervention initiative for grandparents raising grandchildren orphaned by AIDS and one for a study of religious coping among older persons in communities with a high prevalence of HIV/AIDS. The KU-GSU team also is developing plans for a U.S. conference on African aging, in collaboration with the Association for Anthropology and Gerontology and the African Gerontological Society.

TEACHING GERONTOLOGY IN KENYA

Although still in the planning stages, KU's proposed diploma in gerontology has attracted much attention from students and practitioners alike. The rationale and objectives for the gerontology diploma are described as follows in a recent KU report on the progress of the program:

> Currently, there are few and limited training programmes in Kenya that cater to older persons. These programmes are managed by people who are not usually adequately prepared to serve the needs

of older persons. Moreover, with the number of older persons projected to increase, there will be continuous need for trained personnel to work with them. Kenyatta University therefore proposes to fill this gap by offering a programme of study in Gerontology. The proposed multi-disciplinary programme is meant to provide high quality training for people who will directly or indirectly offer services to older persons in order to improve their quality of life. The objectives of the programme are: (1) to impart knowledge and understanding on ageing, (2) to train people in organizations already providing services to older persons, (3) to train new entrants in the area of care of older persons, (4) to undertake a review of studies on ageing in Africa, and (5) to establish a research and documentation center on ageing and equip it with adequate literature. (Kenyatta University, 2004, p. 1)

The KU gerontology diploma would be equivalent to an associate degree in the United States. The diploma requires four semesters of courses, plus a practicum. Each semester, students will register for 7 "units" or courses. At KU, a semester is 14 weeks long, and a unit is 35 contact hours. Although this sounds like an extremely heavy course load by U.S. academic standards, it is not an unusual load for KU students. Plans call for the diploma to be a separate program. Students who add a bachelor's degree to the gerontology diploma will require an additional two years to complete their studies. Both students and individuals working in social services or community development are eligible for the diploma. Table 1 shows the courses that comprise the diploma.

Most U.S. gerontology educators would envy KU's list of courses and might view the diploma program as quite ambitious. However, the number of courses is indicative of the level of commitment KU is investing in gerontology education. The new courses at KU will be taught by 13 full-time faculties in the department of sociology, with assistance from faculty in 10 additional departments. Additional specialists will need to be recruited to help teach some courses.

A critical need for the new program is instructional material. Like many educational institutions in developing countries, Kenyatta University's library resources are limited. The GSU Institute applied for and received a small grant from the African Librarians Council of the African Studies Association to cover mailing costs of gerontology texts and journals to KU. To date, GSU has donated over 300 books and journals to the KU Bureau of Educational Research library. Another source

TABLE 1. Kenyatta University Gerontology Diploma List of Courses

African Social and Cultural Context of Aging	Nutrition and Aging
Family Relations and Aging	Aging and Poverty
Population and Aging	Policy, Legislation, and Aging
Socio-Economic Issues in Aging	Creativity and Aging
Communication and Older Persons	Aging and Disability
Health and the Aging Process	Cultural Diversity and Aging
Aging in Rural and Urban Contexts	Physiology of Aging
Psychology of Aging	Recreation and Leisure for Older Persons
Research Methodology in Gerontology	Ethics and Aging
Theories of Aging	Aging, Crime, and Deviance
Aging, Religion, and Spirituality	Disaster Issues and Older Persons
Gender Issues and Aging	Resource Mobilization and Management
Health Care Delivery for Older Persons	for Older Persons
Sexuality and Aging	Older Persons and Information Technology

of instructional material for KU is electronic media that will enable faculty to download and print electronic gerontology journals and books.

The future of gerontology education in Kenya rests largely, as in the U.S., on the support of the university's administration and future funding opportunities. Fortunately, the Vice Chancellor of Kenyatta University (equivalent to the President or Chancellor of an American university) is supportive of the new program and values gerontology as an academic discipline. KU's new gerontology program also has national support. Dr. Gachuhi and his colleagues endorsed a national policy on older persons, which includes the formation of a National Advisory Council of Older Persons and Aging under the Kenya Department of Social Services. Further, Dr. Gachuhi has established a Coordinating Inter-University Gerontology Research Committee with other educational institutions in Eastern Africa. Efforts also are underway to start a Gerontology Association of Eastern Africa, comprised of the 18 countries in the United Nations' Eastern Africa Region, which would be the third gerontology association on the continent, joining the African Gerontological Society, based in Ghana, and the South African Gerontology and Geriatrics Association, based in Cape Town, South Africa. Plans also are in process to establish an *Eastern Africa Journal of Gerontology*, an official journal of the new Eastern Africa association and an outlet for research papers originating from the region.

CULTURAL COMPETENCE
AND INTERNATIONAL ACADEMIC PARTNERSHIPS

Increasing Cultural Competence

As mutually beneficial as the KU-GSU gerontology partnership has been, it has required both institutions to increase their cultural competence. In her AGHE presentation, Maria Cattell defined cultural competence among international institutions as acquiring an understanding of the international partner's beliefs, values, responsibilities, and relationships in order to enhance the success of collaborative programs (Cattell, 2004). According to Cattell, gerontology educators and students who seek a relationship with institutions in other countries should familiarize themselves with their host country's social customs, academic traditions, and attitudes toward aging. Cattell discussed some of the cultural competence issues she has faced over the past 22 years in her participant observation and longitudinal research among the Luyia ethnic community in rural western Kenya. Her research focused on older persons in their families and communities, including the effects of rapid socioeconomic, technological, political, and cultural change, deepening poverty, and HIV/AIDS on the Kenya family system and the roles of older women and men in Kenyan society (Cattell, 1999; 2002). Among the values and beliefs Dr. Cattell cited as especially important in cross-cultural interactions with Kenyans were: the importance of hospitality; the significance of status, respect, and obedience to those in authority in a patriarchal society; fluid attitudes toward time; and the importance of familiarity.

Experiences with Cultural Competence Issues

Kenyans' adherence to the values referred to by Cattell surfaces in both official and informal interactions, particularly in the academic setting. For example, in Kenyan society, one hears the term *karibu* frequently. It means "welcome," and it is more than a passing expression. Hospitality is a social obligation taken quite seriously in Kenya, as it is in many other African countries. Visitors (especially those from far away) *must* be made to feel welcomed. During their first visit to Kenya, Whittington and King experienced some embarrassment at the "red carpet treatment" they received and the deference paid them by everyone from university administrators to the housekeeping staff at the on-campus residence where they stayed. American scholars may find that the African emphasis on hospitality takes some getting used to. In her AGHE discussion of her medical students' field experiences among elders of the Luo ethnic community (Ice, 2004), Gillian Ice described the formalities observed by the community leaders each time her team arrived in a village. A *twak* or speech was offered by each village leader and selected community members, welcoming Dr. Ice's team and expressing appreciation for the services they provided. At times somewhat lengthy, the welcoming speeches, while appreciated, led to a conflict with Dr. Ice's time constraints, prompting her to preface subsequent visits with the announcement, "No *twak* today, please!"

The GSU team also learned that Kenyan hospitality should be acknowledged and reciprocated by guests in a tangible way. An exchange of gifts was an important first step in solidifying the KU-GSU partnership. During his second visit to Atlanta, Dr. Gachuhi presented the Gerontology Institute with an oil painting of a *kamati ya wazee* (council of elders), along with several colorful kangas (skirts) and gifts of Kenyan coffee and tea. During a welcoming seminar for the GSU team's first visit to Nairobi, Dr. Whittington presented a bronze clock with a GSU insignia to the presiding chair of the seminar, assuming that the chair was the appropriate recipient. What followed was illustrative of another cultural value mentioned by Dr. Cattell–the significance of status and lower–ranking individuals' respect for authority figures. The seminar chair, a faculty member, promptly handed the GSU clock to the Deputy Vice Chancellor (DVC). Later, it was learned that the DVC appropriately presented the clock to the Vice Chancellor, the head of the university, who was unable to attend the seminar. Another opportunity to reciprocate KU's hospitality and provide some well-deserved acknowledgement came during the same seminar when Dr. Whittington presented Dr. Gachuhi with an honorary gerontology certificate from GSU–the same certificate received by graduates of the program.

Another important cultural value, the Kenyan cultural tendency to adopt a fluid attitude toward time (sometimes referred to by Kenyans as "African time"), may cause some discomfort for task-oriented, time-conscious, deadline-driven American academics. Academic meetings and other gatherings have social as well as professional value among Kenyans, and many are less concerned about adhering to strict starting and ending times, as are some Americans. The GSU team learned that the Kenyan cultural value of respect for authority also can affect scheduling of activities. If administrators were scheduled to attend a meeting or event (which, as in the U.S., is very important for academic politics), that event may be delayed significantly until the invited administrator arrives.

Finally, the importance of familiarity in Kenyan culture can be a key factor in establishing an international partnership because of its role in trust-building. Many Americans share this value, particularly in business relationships, and we prefer to do business with individuals or organizations that have followed through reliably on previous transactions. Trust was one of Kenyatta University's paramount concerns in its decision to establish a link with Georgia State. During the first meeting between the GSU team and KU administrators, one of the Deputy Vice Chancellors shared his concerns about previous institutional links that had proved unsatisfying because of the lack of follow-through on the part of the international partner. The point was made that the university did not want to simply "entertain tourists" without realizing any tangible benefits.

The GSU team was appreciative of the Deputy Vice Chancellor's candor, and his comments greatly enhanced the team's awareness of KU's expectations for the relationship. This awareness proved beneficial as the partnership progressed. For example, the GSU team identified a potential funding opportunity that required the inclusion of an additional partner institution from the University System of Georgia. The GSU team proceeded to make the necessary arrangements with another Georgia university and drafted a grant proposal that included GSU, KU, and the new third partner, only to learn that KU was unwilling to participate in a project that involved an unknown institution with whom they had no formal relationship. Although KU later agreed to proceed with the grant application, the importance of familiarity in international relations was made clear to the GSU team.

TALES FROM THE FIELD: THE BENEFITS AND CHALLENGES OF GERONTOLOGY FIELD EDUCATION IN A DEVELOPING COUNTRY

Benefits of Gerontology Field Education

Establishing a working relationship with an academic institution in another part of the world is an exciting undertaking. However, most

Americans experience developing countries from "arm's length," either from images and pictures or as a tourist cushioned from the day-to-day realties of functioning in an environment where many of the conveniences we take for granted are unavailable. The GSU team's visits to several programs for impoverished older adults (which were far outside the "tourist zone" of Nairobi) introduced them to the physical and emotional challenges Americans face if they choose to work at the "grass roots" level in a developing country. Ice (2004) believes that gerontological field training and programming in a developing country is the best way to help students put a face on the term "global aging." In her AGHE presentation, Ice shared her field experiences from her Kenyan Grandparents Study, designed to examine emotional, behavioral, and physiological response to the stress of caregiving and to examine the health outcomes associated with stress among Luo grandparents in rural, western Kenya.

Because the cultural content in medical education often is sporadic and medical students tend to shy away from social and cultural curricula, Ice takes what she calls a "back door" approach to cross-cultural geriatrics education by inviting her students to participate in her research. Medical students can participate under two curricular mechanisms: a Summer Research Fellowship program for 1st year medical students and a research rotation for 3rd and 4th year medical students. During her most recent visit to Kenya, Dr. Ice's team of students interviewed 200 individuals 50 years and older about their caregiving roles and health history and conducted 200 clinical histories and physicals (referred to as H & Ps) in 17 days. A 4th year medical student who participated in the study last year proudly exclaimed, "I've conducted more H&Ps in 17 days than in 2 years of clinical rotations."

Among the benefits Dr. Ice believes the students receive is the clinical experience of observing geriatric health conditions to which they would have little to no exposure in the U.S., such as malaria, brucellosis, filariasis, and bilharzia. Encountering these kinds of health conditions help students develop multiple levels of clinical expertise. In addition, they observe tremendous variation in the aging process, in contrast to some of their perceptions of "normal aging." Additional benefits include understanding and working within the existing health structure, which relies primarily on local healers, the use of traditional medicinal plants, and ritual health practices. For example, students were fascinated by the practice of removing uvulas and ritual scarring. Finally, their fieldwork in an area with one of the highest HIV/AIDS prevalence rates in Kenya gave Dr. Ice's students real-life exposure to the impact of HIV/AIDS on older adults.

Challenges of Gerontology Fieldwork in a Developing Country

Instructional as the students' rotation in Nyanza province was, they faced numerous challenges, including language barriers, adjusting to native foods, the emotional strain of observing severe health conditions for which no solution or treatment was available, and functioning in an impoverished environment. They were distressed at the number of treatable conditions they encountered such as malnutrition, lymphomas, hernias, and anemia. Dr. Ice spoke of one student who was bothered by the numerous flies that swarmed around her as she examined one of the elders. Pulling her hat over her eyes to provide some protection prevented eye contact with the elders she was examining and interviewing. Dr. Ice corrected the student's behavior, which some elders might interpret as disrespectful. Students' motivations for participating in the rotation also influenced their experiences. One of Dr. Ice's African American students signed on for the trip because she "always wanted to travel to Africa." The hard work and difficult conditions she encountered were more than she had bargained for, but the experience became life-changing in ways that she did not expect. One of the students was Kenyan, and the trip provided him an opportunity to return home and visit his grandmother. For Dr. Ice, having a graduate student who was a Kenyan native was a valuable asset. The student was a cultural resource for the whole team. He assisted with translation, acted as a guide, mentored other students, and functioned as an "ambassador" with community leaders. Further, the experience strengthened his resolve to come back and apply the knowledge that he gained in the United States.

According to Ice, the challenges to the field approach to international gerontology education are numerous and difficult, particularly because of dependence on outside funding. Also, "hand-holding" students with varying personalities for several weeks in a developing country, with few "creature comforts" and pronounced cultural differences was, as she described it, a "24-hour job." However, the benefits of the fieldwork can be equally substantial. From an educational perspective, field research experience can stimulate interest in public health, research, and cross-cultural communication–three areas traditionally not of interest to medical students. Students sharpened their skills in cultural competence and communication by applying seemingly abstract classroom concepts. Such a field approach can train people at multiple levels. From the researcher's perspective, students provide an invaluable asset in completing a large research project in a relatively short period. The community benefits by receiving yearly physical exams and health information. Based on her 2003 experience, Ice is now preparing health education materials so that community members can learn to care for themselves and become health advocates for others.

CONCLUSION AND RECOMMENDATIONS

In this article, we have presented an overview of the process of establishing an international gerontology partnership with a Kenyan university and some of the cultural experiences gained and lessons learned through aging research in Kenya. To conclude, we offer several recommendations for gerontology programs interested in forming an international link.

For global aging to become "real" for gerontology educators and students, an investment in an international gerontology partnership–either with an academic institution, an NGO, or community-based group, such as a faith-based program-provides a greater depth of cultural experience and learning than can be achieved by short-term visits to other countries and observations of gerontological or geriatric programs sponsored by other organizations or institutions. An international gerontology partnership (either formal or informal) requires the same delicacy as any meaningful relationship. The process of traversing the "cultural gap" that separates international gerontology partners is itself a source of global aging education, and this process is best achieved in a face-to-face setting. For this reason, the first recommendation for establishing a gerontology partnership is to seek funding for *multiple* visits to the intended partner's country and, if possible, additional funding for an exchange visit of the partner to the United States. The importance of making several visits relates to the cultural value of familiarity and trust-building that is essential for an international relationship to thrive. A single visit, followed by only written or electronic communication, provides limited exposure to the cultural context of the international partner and can project a "tourist" image. As an example, Maria Cattell reported about how emotionally distant some of her western Kenyan informants were, even after she had lived in the area for two years. When she returned two years later to follow up her research, her informants greeted her warmly, hugging her profusely. When she inquired why her informants had not been as affectionate while she was living among them, she was told it was her return after having been away for a time that demonstrated her care for them. Their comment was: "It wasn't until you came back that we knew you really loved us."

Although the ultimate goal of a partnership may be collaborative research or clinical experience, a second recommendation is to provide a service or other material benefit. For example, Dr. Ice's free medical examinations for elders and Dr. King's faculty development workshop helped build trust and strengthened personal and professional ties. In addition to offering services, tangible contributions also are greatly appreciated, such as GSU's book donations.

Our third recommendation is to utilize existing cultural resources. A student who is a native of the proposed partner country, like Dr. Ice's Kenyan student, can greatly facilitate the relationship-building process. Prior to their first visit to KU, the GSU team benefited from discussions with an Atlanta acquaintance of Dr. Gachuhi, a Kenyan business professional whose wife is a graduate of Kenyatta University. Because of his enthusiasm for the KU-GSU partnership, he offered the GSU team valuable insight into day-to-day life in Kenya, cultural traditions, and academic customs and procedures.

Finding "common ground" with an international gerontology partner is our fourth recommendation. For the KU-GSU partnership, the topic of grandparents raising grandchildren linked the two institutions in a very significant way. GSU's own *Project Healthy Grandparents*, a program of the GSU National Center on Grandparents Raising Grandchildren, and the Gerontology Institute's NIA-funded study of religion and health in three-generation African American families provided the impetus for GSU's interest in grand parenting. For KU, the rapidly increasing number of grandparents raising children orphaned by AIDS is a growing concern. This shared interest in older family caregivers emerged during the first meeting between the GSU team and the KU faculty and continues to influence the partnership's emerging research and proposal-writing agenda.

Our fifth recommendation is to identify other gerontology scholars who have conducted research or spent time in the proposed host country. The KU-GSU team's affiliation with Drs. Ice and Cattell has greatly enhanced their partnership with KU. Further, Dr. Ice's fieldwork in the Nyanza province encouraged the GSU team to target that region for the proposed KU-GSU intervention project for grandparent caregivers of orphans. Those seeking international partnerships should inquire about in-country gerontologists, aging advocates, or aging "stakeholders," such as Dr. Gachuhi at KU, who may have done important groundwork. Helpful sources of this information are the International Association of Gerontology, the host country's government social services offices, major international organizations, such as CARE, UNICEF, or CDC, and international programs of U.S. religious organizations.

Finally, when the Peace Corps was created in the 1960s, recruitment advertisements referred to it as "the toughest job you'll ever love"—a phrase which aptly describes international gerontology work. Gerontology professionals willing to invest the time, funds, and energy to establish an international link (and who are willing to vacate their physical, professional, and cultural "comfort zones") are very likely to get more than they bargained for—both in the benefit of an unparalleled cultural learning experience and in the opportunity to provide an immeasurable service to an organization or institution in a developing country. As gerontologists, we know that the whole world is aging. Establishing international gerontology partnerships will help us learn exactly what that means.

REFERENCES

Adamchak, D. J. (1996). Population ageing: Gender, family support and the economic conditions of older Africans. *Southern African Journal of Gerontology, 5(2)*, 3-8.

Akinsola, H. A. (2000). Effects of the AIDS epidemic and the community home-based care programme on the health of older Batswana. *Southern African Journal of Gerontology, 9(1)*, 4-9.

Angel, J. L. (2003). Devolution and the social welfare of elderly immigrants: Who will bear the burden? *Public Administration Review, 63*, 79-89.

Apt, N. (2002a). Preface. In S. Makoni & K. Stroeken (Eds.), *Ageing in Africa: Sociolinguistic and anthropological approaches* (pp. ix-xii). Hampshire, England: Ashgate.

_____(2002b). Ageing and the changing role of the family and the community: An African perspective. *International Social Security Review, 55(1)*, 39-47.

Bailey, C., & Turner, J. (2002). Social security in Africa: A brief overview. *Journal of Aging & Social Policy, 14(1)*, 105-114.

Barresi, C. M., & Stull, D. E. (1993). Ethnicity and long-term care: An overview. In C. M. Barresi & D. E. Stull (Eds.), *Ethnic elderly and long term care* (pp. 3-21). New York: Springer.

Bongaarts, J., & Zimmer, Z. (2002). Living arrangements of older adults in the developing world: An analysis of demographic and health survey household surveys. *Journals of Gerontology, 57B (3)*, S145-S157.

Cattell, M. G. (1999). Gender, aging and health among the Samia of Kenya: A case study. In M. Ferreira, N. Apt, & A. Kirambi (Eds.), *Ageing in changing societies:*

Africa preparing for the next millennium (pp. 106-122). Accra, Ghana: African Gerontological Society.

_____(2002). Holding up the sky: Gender, age and work among Abaluyia of Kenya. In S. Makoni & K. Stroeken (Eds.), *Ageing in Africa: Sociolinguistic and anthropological approaches* (pp. 157-177). Hampshire, England: Ashgate.

_____(2004). Cultural Competence in western Kenya: Implications for gerontology research and education. A paper presented at the Annual Meeting of the Association of Gerontology in Higher Education, Richmond, February, 2004.

Eke, B. (2003). Impact of AIDS on intergenerational relationships in Africa. *Journal of Intergenerational Relationships, 1(3)*, 9-24.

Fenech, F. F. (2002). Second world assembly on aging. *Bold, 12(4)*, p. 3-5.

Ferreira, M. (1999). Building and advancing African gerontology. Editorial. *Southern African Journal of Gerontology, 8*, 1-3.

_____(2000). Growing old in the new South Africa. *Ageing International, 25(4)*, 32-46.

Ferreira, M., & Makoni, S. (1999). Does Alzheimer's disease occur in Africans? *Africa Health, 21*, 14-15.

_____(2002). Towards a cultural and linguistic construction of late-life dementia in an urban African population. In S. Makoni & K. Stroeken (Eds.), *Ageing in Africa: Sociolinguistic and anthropological approaches* (pp. 21-41). Hampshire, England: Ashgate.

Gachuhi, M. (2004). Establishing national and international inter-university collaboration in research and curriculum development in gerontology. A paper presented at the Annual Meeting of the Association of Gerontology in Higher Education, Richmond, February, 2004.

Gorman, J. (2000). Growing problem of violence against older persons in Africa. *Southern African Journal of Gerontology, 9(2)*, 33-36.

Ice, G. (2004). Gerontological education in the field. A paper presented at the Annual Meeting of the Association of Gerontology in Higher Education, Richmond, February, 2004.

Ineichen, B. (2000). Epideminiology of dementia in Africa: A review. *Social Science and Medicine, 50*, 1673-1677.

International HIV/AIDS Alliance & HelpAge International (2003). *Forgotten families: Older people as carers of orphans and vulnerable children.* Brighton, England: International HIV/AIDS Alliance.

Joubert, J., & Lindgren, P. (2003). HEAL: An intervention project addressing elder abuse in South Africa. *Intercom, 10(3)*, 4-6.

Kenyatta University. (2004). Kenyatta University diploma in gerontology: Study of Ageing Process. A report presented at the Kenyatta University Gerontology Induction Workshop, Nairobi, May, 24, 2004.

Kinsella, K., & Velkoff, V. A. (2001). *An aging world: 2001.* U.S. Census Bureau Series 95/01-1. Washington, DC: U.S. Government Printing Office.

Lloyd, S. P. (2002). Formal social protection for older people in developing countries: Three different approaches. *Journal of Social Policy, 31(4)*, 695-713.

Makoni, S., & Stroeken, K. (2002). Towards transdisciplinary studies on ageing in Africa. In S. Makoni & K. Stroeken (Eds.), *Ageing in Africa: Sociolinguistic and anthropological approaches* (pp. 1-18). Hampshire, England: Ashgate.

Mba, C. J. (2003). Living arrangements of the elderly women of Lesotho. *Bold, 14(1)*, 3-20.

Van der Geest, S. (2002). From wisdom to witchcraft: Ambivalence towards old age in rural Ghana. *Africa, 72(3)*, 437-463.

Williams, A. (2003). *Ageing and poverty in Africa: Ugandan livelihoods in a time of HIV/AIDS*. Hampshire, England: Ashgate.

Wilson, A. O., & Adamchak, D. J. (2001). Grandmother's disease: The impact of AIDS on Africa's older women. *Age and Ageing, 30(1)*, 8-10.

Teaching Chinese Health Care Professionals About Community-Based Long-Term Care in China

Bei Wu, PhD

SUMMARY. Academic exchanges between the U.S. and other countries around the world are increasing and teaching students abroad is part of this trend. China is in its initial stage of developing gerontology education and is in great need of new concepts and ideas for dealing with its rapidly aging population. This paper discusses the challenges and rewards of teaching gerontology to health care professionals in China. To achieve the desired learning outcomes in another country requires culturally appropriate course materials and teaching methods; drawing on students' knowledge and expertise by using an interactive format and gaining students' respect. *[Article copies available for a fee from The Haworth Document Delivery Service: 1-800-HAWORTH. E-mail address: <docdelivery@haworthpress.com> Website: <http://www.HaworthPress.com> © 2005 by The Haworth Press, Inc. All rights reserved.]*

KEYWORDS. Cultural exchange, culturally-appropriate materials, teaching methods, elder-care in China, community-based long-term care, academic gerontology

---

Bei Wu is Assistant Professor, West Virginia University, Center on Aging and Department of Community Medicine, P.O. Box 9127, Morgantown, WV 26506 (E-mail: bwu@hsc.wvu.edu).

[Haworth co-indexing entry note]: "Teaching Chinese Health Care Professionals About Community-Based Long-Term Care in China." Wu, Bei. Co-published simultaneously in *Gerontology & Geriatrics Education* (The Haworth Press, Inc.) Vol. 26, No. 1, 2005, pp. 137-149; and: *Aging Education in a Global Context* (ed: Dena Shenk, and Lisa Groger) The Haworth Press, Inc., 2005, pp. 137-149. Single or multiple copies of this article are available for a fee from The Haworth Document Delivery Service [1-800- HAWORTH, 9:00 a.m. - 5:00 p.m. (EST). E-mail address: docdelivery@haworthpress.com].

The elder care support system in China has recently received attention because of the dramatic increase of China's older population. China is in great need of new concepts and ideas for dealing with its rapidly aging population and the profound impact this population is having on socio-economic development. Selected as a teaching fellow by the Overseas Young Chinese Forum (OYCF), I taught a short-term course on community-based long-term care (CBLTC) for elders to health care professionals at the Shanghai University Sociology Department. OYCF is a U.S.-based policy oriented nonprofit organization that is interested in funding teaching and research in China. I am a bilingual and bicultural professor at a U.S. academic institution, and conducted research on aging in China for several years in the late 1980s and early 1990s. The purpose of the course was to introduce U.S. and European models of CBLTC to Chinese health care professionals and to provide them with insights into how best to develop China's long-term care system.

BACKGROUND

China has a tradition of caring for elders at home, with responsibility for frail elders falling exclusively on family members—mainly spouses or adult children. These arrangements based on traditional expectations of filial responsibility worked well in pre-industrial China. However, demographic changes and recent economic developments have had a profound impact on the traditional family and its support system, making it increasingly more difficult for family members to meet the ideal and fulfill the cultural expectation of caring for their elders.

Impact of China's Demographic Changes

China has experienced significant change in the size and proportion of older adults over the past two decades, and this trend will continue for the next 50 years (Zeng, Vaupel, Xiao, & Liu, 2002). China's elder population, defined as adults aged 60 years and older, reached 130 million in 2000 and comprised more than 10% of the total population. The oldest-old, those aged 80 years and older, grew to approximately 11.5 million in 2000 and accounted for nearly 9% of all elders aged 60 years and older (National Bureau of Statistics of China, 2002). By 2020, China's population aged 60 years and older is estimated to reach 243 million representing 17% of the total population (National Population and Family Planning Commission of China, 2003). In addition to growing in absolute numbers, the aged population in China is expected to undergo significant aging itself. It is estimated that the number of the oldest-old will reach 27.80 million in 2020 (Yue, 2001).

The rapid growth of China's aging population in absolute terms and as a percentage of the total population is largely due to the implementation of the one child policy over the last two decades coupled with a sizable increase in average life expectancy (Harbaugh & West, 1993; Yuan, Zhang, Ping, Li, & Liang, 1992). Due to smaller families with fewer children, the availability of family members to provide care and support to their older parents will most likely continue to decrease (Bartlett & Phillips, 1997).

Impact of Economic Reform

Economic factors have affected individual filial piety, values, economic status, living conditions, and living arrangements of elders and their families in several ways. First, working adult children may find it more difficult than in the past to take care of their frail parents because recent improvements in housing conditions have increased the likelihood that adult children have their own apartments and live separately from their parents. This greater independence of adult children from their elders raises concerns about care when elders become frail. The problems created by separate living arrangements are further exacerbated by the growing geographic mobility of younger adults in China. Economic developments have created attractive job opportunities for young adults, but those opportunities may not be located where their parents live.

Second, more people can afford to purchase labor outside of their home for elder care. Therefore, although most adult children still consider it their responsibility to provide care for older parents, they are increasingly looking for ways to assist them in caring for their elders as they struggle to fulfill their multiple competing responsibilities.

Development of Community-Based Long-Term Care in China

One response to the concerns and challenges of caring for current and future elders has been the growth of nursing homes. Nursing home care for the old and frail is becoming an increasingly common but expensive option in China. While nursing home care is an option for the sickest and most disabled, it may be an unrealistic option for all elders in need of care. Instead, various forms of CBLTC services and programs have begun to emerge in China, especially in more densely populated, urban centers. As used in this paper, the concept of community-based services and programs refers to a set of care services such as personal care, homemakers, and adult day care, which are delivered to frail elders in their community. The demand for community-based services and programs for elders has become a critical issue in China.

In response to this need, more jobs for *bao mu* (literally, housemaids) have been created to meet the needs of elders. *Bao mu* provide various in-home services for elders and their families, sometimes caring simultaneously for younger children and older grandparents. Many private service coordination centers have been established to serve as intermediate placement agencies for elders and *bao mu* (Wu, Carter, Goins, & Cheng, in press).

In addition, since 2000, the Shanghai Civil Affairs Bureau has required every street committee (*Jie Dao*) to establish a community service center and has invested money at each district level for the construction of such a center. The purpose of these centers is to provide services to meet their clients' daily needs, with elders being the recipients of most services. As a result of this initiative, the vast majority of street committees currently have a community service center. However, few of these centers have their own personnel or staff to provide direct services. The vast majority of the centers serve as clearinghouses for home care services, that is, community residents request services and the center matches them with registered service providers. The centers are not responsible for price negotiations or for determining what types of services should be provided.

Efforts to develop new models of CBLTC for elders in China have received growing attention. Since China is in its initial stage of development of its CBLTC system, many issues need to be addressed regarding training of the workforce, implementation of quality management systems, and increasing investment in the field (see Wu et al., in press), for a detailed description of policy implications for improving the current CBLTC in China. The U.S. and Europe started developing CBLTC systems several decades ago. Although these systems may not be perfect and could probably be improved in many ways, China can learn from the experiences of Western countries, especially as they relate to the initial stage of the development of such systems.

Gerontological Education in China

Gerontology education in China did not begin until the 1980s. The primary emphasis of China's gerontology programs has been research, not education. Thus the growth of gerontology education has historically lagged behind that of gerontology research. During the past decade, more universities began offering gerontology courses in several disciplines. However, the aging-related programs at most universities that offer such courses focus only on their own discipline (e.g., sociology, psychology, social work, and economics); there is a lack of collaboration and interaction between the disciplines. More multidisciplinary gerontology programs and courses need to be developed. To-date, the development of gerontology education has not met the needs of Chinese professionals or the older population. Given the tremendous size of the older population, many service organizations for elders, such as residential care facilities and CBLTC facilities, have been established, not all of which are government-sponsored institutions. There has been an uncharacteristic increase in the number of privately-owned organizations serving elders (Wu et al., in press), but very few service providers who work in the field have been trained in gerontology. Therefore, gerontology education in China needs to be developed on two levels: to expand training for future professionals who intend to work with elders, and to provide continuing gerontology education to eldercare professionals who are currently providing care to elders. Given the need for gerontology education for professionals in China, the purpose of this paper is to identify ways for improving teaching methodologies to be used not only with Chinese health care providers, but that can be applied to other settings as well.

TEACHING AT SHANGHAI UNIVERSITY

In 2002, I received a teaching fellowship from the OYCF to teach a short-term, policy-related CBLTC course in the Shanghai University Sociology Department. This course was part of a one-time Sociology graduate certificate program jointly sponsored by the Shanghai University Sociology Department and the Shanghai Civil Affairs Bureau. The Municipal Civil Affairs Bureau is a government organization which is in charge of social welfare. The bureau conducts and disseminates policy-relevant research on issues related to aging and community-based care. The objectives of the graduate certificate program were to provide staff (most of whom were employed by health care service agencies) with the opportunity for continuing education, and to improve the quality of the workforce serving elders. In addition to the course I taught, the program offered nine other courses: Introduction to Sociology, Fundamentals of Sociology, Family Sociology, Social Work, Social Psychology, Survey Methods, Social Welfare, Sociological Theories in Western Countries, and Statistics. Thus, my policy course was the only aging-related course in the Sociology Certificate Program.

Part-time graduate students employed in organizations affiliated with the Shanghai Civil Affairs Bureau were enrolled in my policy course. The 32 students enrolled in the course included administrators from local civil affairs offices and committees on aging, heads of residential care facilities, and administrators from mental health hospitals.

Course Objectives

The course met for six hours a week for four weeks in December 2002. The objectives of the course were to provide students with a basic understanding of major current CBLTC arrangements in the U.S. and of developments of CBLTC in China, and to carry out an analysis of a significant long-term care policy issue in China.

Course Content and Format

The course used a combination of lectures and class discussion. Stone's (2000) report helped shape the outline for the course. The first half of the course introduced CBLTC systems and policies in the U.S. and introduced the main topics: definition and history of long-term care; long-term care financing; long-term care service delivery; long-term care workforce; and the future of long-term care demand and supply. Specifically, I described several successful models and programs of community-based long-term care in the U.S. but also identified the shortcomings of the CBLTC system in the US.

The remainder of the class was devoted to discussions of the current state of long-term care in China and to what extent China can learn from the U.S. experience for developing its own long-term care system. As many students had first-hand knowledge of the Chinese long-term care system, they actively participated in class discussions. Discussions focused on policy and practical implications for developing long-term care in China.

Reading Materials

Reading materials were chosen from multiple sources. The readings in Chinese discussed the Chinese and/or U.S. long-term care systems. I selected these materials from my personal collection of Chinese books and journal papers, Chinese websites, and papers and books from interlibrary loans. Having been a researcher at Shanghai Research Center on Aging ten years earlier and having maintained a close relationship with Chinese in the field of aging, I remain informed of developments in gerontology in China. As a board member of the Shanghai Research Center on Aging, I often receive books and journals from colleagues in China. Reading materials also included articles in English on the U.S. long-term care system and China's support system. Given the fact that most of the students had a limited command of English, most required reading materials were in Chinese.

Class Assignments

Students were required to conduct field visits and to interview two or three administrators from local community service centers. I designed a survey instrument for the students to use in their interviews that covered several dimensions: (1) demographic information of the organization; (2) current long-term care services provided by the organization; (3) workforce issues; and (4) interviewee's job satisfaction. The instrument design was based on the literature about CBLTC in the U.S. and China and on class discussion. In the end, students interviewed administrators from 64 different community organizations that serve elders in Shanghai. These organizations included community-service centers and residential care facilities that recently extended their functions to provide day-care to elders in the community. Students were required to write a policy paper based on readings, class discussion and their field interviews.

CHALLENGES OF TEACHING THE COURSE

Many challenges emerged during the process of preparing the course syllabus and subsequently teaching the course. This was the first time I had taught such a course, although I had conducted research projects on this topic (Wu, 2000, Wu & Emerson Lombardo, 2000). Although I had no language problem in teaching this course, this was the first time I taught a course in a Chinese setting since I came to the U.S. a decade earlier. Below I describe some of the specific challenges I encountered in preparing and teaching the course.

Lack of Appropriate Reading Materials

One of the main problems was the lack of appropriate reading materials. Although English language skills have improved greatly among young college and graduate students in China in the past decade, most nontraditional students still have quite limited English language skills. I was aware of this issue during the process of designing the course and therefore required students to read only one or two papers in English, with additional papers in English being optional.

To enable students to grasp the course content in a reasonable amount of time, most required readings were in Chinese. However, the lack of Chinese materials on the subject was a serious issue. As stated earlier, caring for frail elders has traditionally almost exclusively been provided by family members. Institutional support and CBLTC are only in the initial stages of development. As a result, Chinese literature on this topic is scarce. Most available literature pointed out the challenges to family support for elders (Gao, 2003; Xu, 2003; Yao, 2002; Yao, Xu, Zeng & Fang, 1997). Policy implications for long-term care systems resulting from these studies were broad-based, vague attempts at a macro level analysis and lacked any empirical underpinnings. Furthermore, there is even less literature available in Chinese translation of materials that introduce U.S. or European long-term care systems. Thus, my students had to rely heavily on lectures to gain an understanding of the CBLTC system in the U.S. It was a challenge for me to create succinct and, at the same time, comprehensive lectures given the complexity of the CBLTC system in the U.S.

Interpreting English Terms

Terms that are quite common in gerontology in the U.S, such as Medicare, Medicaid, Supplemental Security Income (SSI), Activity of Daily Living (ADL), and Instrumental Activity of Daily Living (IADL), are not familiar to many people in China. Most of these terms have been translated, and I had to be very careful to use terms consistent with existing Chinese translations with which the students were familiar. Using different terms would have been confusing to students who might have thought the terms referred to different programs or concepts.

Instructor Perceived as an "Outsider"

Another challenge I faced was the need to establish myself as an "expert" and "insider" in the eyes of my students. The students enrolled in the class were non-traditional; most of them were experienced administrators working in the health care field and had first-hand experience and knowledge about long-term care in China. Although I had conducted research on aging in Shanghai for several years and still know many people in the aging network in Shanghai, I have since spent a decade in the U.S. and am currently working at a U.S. academic institution. Thus, at the beginning of the course some students still regarded me as an outsider. As a result of this perception of me as an outsider, some were reluctant to speak freely on current issues of the long-term care system in China.

Instructor Not Perceived as an "Authority"

My age and gender were also challenging issues. Most students in the class were male and older than myself. Traditionally, older males are often perceived as authority figures in Chinese society (Fei, 1985). It was a challenge for me as a female who was also younger than most of the students to establish myself as an authority figure in the class. For example, students thought I was familiar only with the U.S. system and did not have updated knowledge and experience on the current state of the elder-care system in China. It was not easy for me to walk into the classroom and lecture my students on a subject that they thought they knew more about than I did. Consequently, some students never did fully engage in discussions.

MEETING THE CHALLENGES

To overcome these barriers and problems, I used multiple methods. For instance, I devoted a great deal of time gaining more first-hand knowledge about China's long-term care system. I also made it clear to my students that I learned from them, and I let them know that their opinions, knowledge and experiences were important. I created an interactive learning environment by devoting class time to open and frank discussion of the issues and policies surrounding long-term care in China.

During the course, I became more familiar with China's recent development of a CBLTC system by conducting field trips and reading policy-related documents and literature. I visited eight representative community-based agencies for CBLTC, including nursing homes that provided CBLTC services in addition to their residential-based services, interviewed policy-makers, government officials and researchers. I also met several officials from the Shanghai Civil Affairs Bureau and researchers from Shanghai University and the Shanghai Research Center on Aging. I had extensive conversations with these native experts on the current state of CBLTC, current issues, and their visions for future development. In addition, I read many documents provided by government officials concerning policy issues in developing a long-term care system in China.

Conducting these activities outside of the classroom made me more knowledgeable about the current state of the long-term care system and more aware of the issues involved. These activities and the additional knowledge I gained helped guide class discussions more appropriately, and to use the reading materials, combined with my first-hand experience, to compensate for some of the gaps in the existing teaching materials.

At the end of the course, one student (the head of the largest residential care facility for elders in Shanghai) told me that he was impressed that I knew so much about China's long-term care policy and system. Most likely, this was the biggest compliment I could have received.

I was aware that it might be difficult to establish myself as an "authority" figure in this class. Therefore, in the classroom, I acknowledged that there is no single authority and that some of my students may know more about the Chinese system than I do. Through this approach, it became clear to my students that through their participation and sharing of ideas, they could make valuable contributions to the course. The friendly and respectful classroom environment I was able to create encouraged students to ask questions, share their knowledge, and fully engage in discussions.

Initially, students struggled with some of the concepts and issues but were able to grasp them better by formulating and working through questions such as: What suggestions would you make to encourage the government's current low investment in CBLTC? How would you effectively allocate limited public funding for long-term care institutions? What kinds of training should frontline workers receive? What would you do to improve the quality of care provided in the community? The class then centered all discussions on trying to answer these questions.

This method of approaching the material made the students more aware of the issues and encouraged and empowered them to make policy recommendations they might not have been able to think of before.

COURSE EVALUATION AND OUTCOMES

Students thought the course was timely, significant, and informative. In terms of the teaching methods, students liked the interactive format and thought this to be an effective way of learning. One student wrote "I particularly like the interactive teaching. This is the first time I have experienced this way of learning in the classroom." Many students thought the method was "creative."

Some students thought the course should have been longer. They would have liked more reading materials in Chinese and to learn more about the current state of CBLTC in the U.S. and Europe. However, due to time constraints this was not possible.

Based on conversations with the students and on class evaluations, indications are that the course had a direct impact on the students' daily work. For example, one student, who is an administrator in a residential care facility, told me that she will add more ethics education to her staff training so that they might be more respectful of elders' rights and privacy. In addition, students made some concrete and insightful suggestions for improving the CBLTC in China. For example, they suggested establishing a tax incentive mechanism for private donations; standardized training for frontline workers; advocating volunteerism in the society; and creating private, nonprofit eldercare service delivery organizations.

CONCLUSIONS

There is an increasing trend toward academic exchanges between the U.S. and other countries around the world. Teaching students abroad is a part of this trend. This paper provides an example of a successful model for teaching health care professionals in China by illustrating that the achievement of course objectives in another country requires multiple considerations. Depending on the experience and educational levels of the students, instructors should develop appropriate teaching methods to fit the special needs of students. Using various ways of drawing upon students' native knowledge and experiences enriches the classroom experience and helps yield optimal results. More importantly, in-structors should be conscientious of how to develop appropriate course materials and teaching methods to enable students to draw on course knowledge derived from other countries and apply these insights to their own country. Instructors need to make an effort to become knowl-edgeable about the host country's culture and subject matter to be sure to communicate materials in a meaningful manner. Instructors' willing-ness to learn relevant aspects for teaching in the host country and a re-spectful attitude towards their students will have a positive impact on the classroom environment. Cultural awareness on the part of the instructor will help gain students' respect, thus assuring good course outcomes.

REFERENCES

Bartlett, H., & Phillips, D.R. (1997). Ageing and aged care in the People's Republic of China: National and local issues and perspectives. *Health & Place*, 3(3), 149-159.

Fei, X.T. (1985). Peasants' Life in China. Beijing: San Lian Publisher.

Gao, H.R. (2003). Current new problems on supporting the aged in the rural families. *Northwest Population Journal*, 3, 34-37.

Harbaugh, C.W., & West, L.A. (1993). Aging trends–China. *Journal of Cross-Cultural Gerontology*, 8, 271-280.

National Bureau of Statistics of China (2002). [Chinese] Retrieved on May 31, 2003, from *http://www.stats.gov.cn/tjfx/ztfx/zgsnrjzs/200206280067.htm*

National Population and Family Planning Commission of China (2003). [Chinese] Re-trieved on April 27, 2004, from *http://www.sfpc.gov.cn/cn/data/sfpcdata2004-1-30-1.htm*

Stone, R. (2000). Long-Term Care for the Elderly with Disabilities: Current Policy, Emerging Trends and Implications for the Twenty-First Century. Milbank Memo-rial Fund. August, 2000.

Wu, B., Carter, M.W., Goins, R.T., & Cheng, C.R. (in press). Emerging services for community-based long-term care (CBLTC) in urban China: A systematic analysis of Shanghai's community-based agencies. *Journal of Aging & Social Policy*, 17, 4.

Wu, B. (2000). *Supplementing Informal Care of Frail Elders with Formal Services: A Comparison of White, Hispanics, and Asian Non-Spousal Caregivers*. Dissertation. University of Massachusetts Boston, Gerontology Program.

Wu, B., & Emerson, N.L. (2000). Serving persons with dementia and their families in the Chinese community: Creative care. *World Alzheimer Congress 2000, Proceed-ings Book*. Washington DC.

Xu, X.J. (2003). Crisis for family support models among empty-nest family in rural ar-eas. Retrieved May 4, 2003, from *http://www.ccrs.org.cn*

Yao, Y., Xu, Q., Zeng, Y., & Fang, H.L. (1997). How far the rural old family support can go? *Population and Development Forum*, 42-50.

Yao, Y.M. (2002). A study of the habitation arrangement of the rural elderly and the quality of life in the Yangtze River Delta. *Journal of Zhejiang University (Humanities and Social Sciences)*, 32(6), 20-26.

Yuan, T.H., Zhang, T., Ping, Y., Li, J., & Liang, Z. (1992). China's demographic dilemmas. *Population Bulletin*, 47, 1-44.

Yue, S.D. (2001). The trend of population aging in China. [Chinese] *Social Security System*, 5.

Zeng, Y, Vaupel, J. W., Xiao, Z. Y., & Liu, Y. Z. (2002). Sociodemographic and health profiles of the oldest old in China. *Population and Development Review*, 28(2): 251-273.

Index

Numbers followed by "f" indicate figures; "t" following a page number indicates tabular material.

151

BOOK ORDER FORM!

Order a copy of this book with this form or online at:
http://www.haworthpress.com/store/product.asp?sku=5719

Aging Education in a Global Context

____ in softbound at $19.95 ISBN-13: 978-0-7890-3081-8 / ISBN-10: 0-7890-3081-0.
____ in hardbound at $39.95 ISBN-13: 978-0-7890-3080-1 / ISBN-10: 0-7890-3080-2.

COST OF BOOKS ____

POSTAGE & HANDLING ____
US: $4.00 for first book & $1.50
for each additional book
Outside US: $5.00 for first book
& $2.00 for each additional book.

SUBTOTAL ____

In Canada: add 7% GST. ____

STATE TAX ____
CA, IL, IN, MN, NJ, NY, OH, PA & SD residents
please add appropriate local sales tax.

FINAL TOTAL ____
If paying in Canadian funds, convert
using the current exchange rate,
UNESCO coupons welcome.

❑ BILL ME LATER:
Bill-me option is good on US/Canada/
Mexico orders only; not good to jobbers,
wholesalers, or subscription agencies.

❑ **Signature** ____

❑ **Payment Enclosed: $** ____

❑ **PLEASE CHARGE TO MY CREDIT CARD:**
❑ Visa ❑ MasterCard ❑ AmEx ❑ Discover
❑ Diner's Club ❑ Eurocard ❑ JCB

Account # ____

Exp Date ____

Signature ____
(Prices in US dollars and subject to change without notice.)

PLEASE PRINT ALL INFORMATION OR ATTACH YOUR BUSINESS CARD

Name ____

Address ____

City ____ State/Province ____ Zip/Postal Code ____

Country ____

Tel ____ Fax ____

E-Mail ____

May we use your e-mail address for confirmations and other types of information? ❑ Yes ❑ No We appreciate receiving
your e-mail address. Haworth would like to e-mail special discount offers to you, as a preferred customer.
We will never share, rent, or exchange your e-mail address. We regard such actions as an invasion of your privacy.

Order from your **local bookstore** or directly from
The Haworth Press, Inc. 10 Alice Street, Binghamton, New York 13904-1580 • USA
Call our toll-free number (1-800-429-6784) / Outside US/Canada: (607) 722-5857
Fax: 1-800-895-0582 / Outside US/Canada: (607) 771-0012
E-mail your order to us: orders@haworthpress.com

For orders outside US and Canada, you may wish to order through your local
sales representative, distributor, or bookseller.
For information, see http://haworthpress.com/distributors

(Discounts are available for individual orders in US and Canada only, not booksellers/distributors.)

Please photocopy this form for your personal use.
www.HaworthPress.com

BOF05